Building Character

T0355730

Building Character

THE ART
AND SCIENCE
OF CASTING

Amy Cook

University of Michigan Press
Ann Arbor

Published in the United States of America by the

University of Michigan Press

Printed and bound by CPI Group (UK) Ltd, Croydon, CR0 4YY

2021   2020   2019   2018   4   3   2   1

A CIP catalog record for this book is available from the British Library.

Library of Congress Cataloging-in-Publication data has been applied for.

ISBN 978-0-472-07376-4 (hardcover : alk. paper)
ISBN 978-0-472-05376-6 (paper : alk. paper)
ISBN 978-0-472-12358-2 (e-book)

Acknowledgments

With each passing year, the list of people to whom I am indebted grows longer. Let me thank and blame all of the following people for inspiring me to finish this project; without the need to thank all of you in print, I might have given up.

When Mark Turner told me after my paper at the Conceptual Structure, Discourse, and Language Conference in Vancouver in 2012, "that's your next book," I should have known better than to think it would be something I could do in a year or two. Luckily, Mark did not just drive-by champion the idea or my work, but remained a mentor and colleague. A man who exhausts the limits of the word indefatigable, I am forever in his debt. I am also grateful to Barbara Dancygier, Eve Sweetser, and Seana Coulson for their insight and inspirational work. Eve welcomed me into her home for a gestures working group while I was on leave in Berkeley, demonstrating what the height of scholarship, collegiality, and hosting looks like.

I was in Berkeley thanks to a grant from Indiana University's College of Arts and Humanities Institute. IU also provided a wealth of brilliant, helpful colleagues—Fritz Breithaupt, Colin Allen, Linda Charnes, Ellen MacKay, Ron Wainscott, and Fontaine Syer, among others. I also had the good fortune to take part in the first few years of *The Albert Wertheim Seminar in Performance*. I am grateful to the contributions made by many smart graduate students at IU, but I have to single out Neal Utterback and Sara Taylor for insights on this project. Neal seemed to take early versions of these thoughts seriously and made me think I should do it before he did. I once asked Sara to help me think through a metaphoric muddle I had gotten myself into, and she gamely rescued me.

I am grateful to Stony Brook University for support through

the Faculty in the Arts, Humanities, and Social Sciences initiative and for a Presidential Travel Grant.

Sections of this book have been published in slightly different versions in books: *The Oxford Handbook of Dance and Theater*, edited by Nadine George-Graves, *Shakespeare and Consciousness*, edited by Paul Budra and Clifford Werier, and *Blending and the Study of Narrative* by Ralf Schneider and Marcus Hartner. Daniel Sack at *Theatre Journal* shaped my review of dreamthinkspeak's *Absent*. The work is better for all their work. Richard Gerrig generously read sections for psychological accuracy and also helped with rhetorical clarity.

Margaret and Donald Freeman hosted me for a short-stay research retreat at the glorious Myrifield Institute for Cognition and the Arts, where they stoked my literal and figurative fire. Margaret continued to provide editorial insight and probing questions. Jessica Landaw also hosted a short-study in her New York apartment, where I could feed only myself and work as many hours in a row as I could stand.

I also want to thank Andrew Sofer; colleagues at the Cognitive Futures in the Arts and Humanities Conferences (especially John Sutton, Seth Frey, Naomi Rokotnitz, and Ellen Spolsky) and the Cognitive Science in Theatre, Dance, and Performance working group at the American Society for Theatre Research conference (especially Rhonda Blair, John Lutterbie, Rick Kemp, Nicola Shaughnessy, and Evelyn Tribble); Dan Irving; David Rodriguez, Kristin Leadbetter; the incomparable LeAnn Fields; Kate Babbitt; and Ken Weitzman, for the cover idea, for creating the character of Donna, and for his many important insights that I probably just assumed were mine.

There are many who fed me, loved me, and put up with me that should be thanked, but it is to Nicole O'Hay that I am forced to dedicate this book because she had to go and die while I was finishing it.

Contents

INTRODUCTION
Character Building

As I walk through the city, the people around me flock and flow. We are a murmuration of starlings: though we are multicolored and multishaped, we are more clearly identifiable as a mass than as individuals. So how is it that we come to identify so many different people in our lives? My doctor, my coworker, and my senator look more alike than different, and yet I do not confuse them because they are *characters* in my life, not data. How do we build characters from stimuli? This book argues that we build the characters of others from a sea of stimuli and that the process of watching actors take on roles improves our ability to "cast" those roles in our daily lives. When it is necessary to make quick judgments about the swarm of those around us, we cast them into categories in order to respond to them more efficiently. The cognitive process that allows us to see Meryl Streep as Margaret Thatcher is the same one that understands Margaret Thatcher as the prime minister or experiences the people murmuring with me on 57th Street as villains, victims, and witnesses.

To cast means many things: to throw, to toss, to fling, to contrive, to reckon, to condemn, to glance. Forty-seven definitions in the *Oxford English Dictionary* precede the theatrical meaning: "to allot (the parts of the play) to the actors." The other definitions are all active; they are about a forceful projection of one thing (a line, an accusation, a head or an eye, a seed) to another (into the water, into jail, onto the ground, down, away). Casting a role is also active; it is a performative act in the sense that characters come to life once they are cast. Hurling an actor into a role creates a character. A casting director may match the perceived qualities of an actor with the perceived qualities of the character, but the combination is also synergistic; casting a character creates qualities. While casting directors do this professionally, all of us do this when we make sense of the people around us. Although we usually think of character building as a process whereby a person comes to have more character due to difficult experiences, the process of building character—our own and those of the figures we see on stage, screen, and life—is one in which human beings "cast" information from one domain to the other, building up layers of meaning in a networked assemblage of bodies, histories, biases, actions, and words. While this book starts with the kind of celebrity casting that can be most visible, it ends with the ways we cast and miscast each other and ourselves.

We are deeply affected by casting. If I said "the man watched the woman," there is no story. If I said, "the man, played by Jack Nicholson, watched the woman," that is a very different story than if I said "the man, played by Matt Damon, watched the woman" or "the man watched the woman, played by Jennifer Lopez." The bodies of the actors—and all that is primed and evoked for us with that body—floods our mind, suggesting the story, leading us to create history and context and to anticipate what is coming next. We may say that an actor is "perfect" for a part or that someone "doesn't look like a doctor," but we know very little about the process that makes one person "right" and another person "wrong." This, in part, is my interest here: the relationship between characters and the bodies that are chosen to represent them. Ultimately, my interest is in the cognitive ability to create characters through casting. What can we learn about how we understand each other and ourselves by examining the casting we find on stage and film—the casting we find perfect and the casting we find wrong?

A massive hack into the Sony Studios computer system in

November 2014 revealed, among other things, that executives at Sony had been discussing the possibility of casting Idris Elba as the next James Bond.[1] A character created in 1953 by Ian Fleming, James Bond has been portrayed by thirteen different actors in many different films. Even when Daniel Craig uttered the words "Bond, James Bond" forty-four years after Sean Connery first did, no one questioned the new iteration. But Idris Elba is black. For some, this was a long-awaited change and for others it was a monstrous idea. Facebook immediately created a "We Want Idris Elba for James Bond" page (which currently has over 35,000 likes), various stars weighed in on the choice (Kanye West and Mindy Kaling are both in favor of this casting), and Rush Limbaugh weighed in on December 23 with his casting expertise:

> James Bond was invented, created by Ian Fleming, a former spy, MI6, and James Bond is a total concept put together by Ian Fleming. He was white and Scottish, period. That is who James Bond is, and I know it's racist to probably even point this out. We had 50 years of white Bonds because Bond is white. Bond was never black. Ian Fleming never created a black Brit to play James Bond. The character was always white. He was always Scottish. He always drank vodka shaken not stirred and all that.[2]

Limbaugh then continues, tongue in cheek, to come up with other casting choices to help Sony "get with the 21st Century" because "we need to be equal" and "we need to be fair about this." He argued, *reductio ad absurdum*, that if Elba played Bond, perhaps George Clooney should play Obama, Kelsey Grammer should play Nelson Mandela, and Rob Reiner should play Al Sharpton. Limbaugh acknowledged that "admittedly, all these characters I've mentioned are real-life characters, and James Bond has never lived, per se, he's a fictional character. But he was white and Scottish."[3] For Limbaugh, the whiteness of Bond's skin and his Scottish heritage is an essential part of who the character is and thus these must be essential traits of the actor cast to play James Bond.[4] Yet Limbaugh did not object to Daniel Day-Lewis, an Irishman, playing Abraham Lincoln, someone for whom being American was a central, if not a visible, part of him.

I realize trotting out Rush Limbaugh's take on this casting choice provides me with a fairly clear straw man, but he was not alone in his views in the online dialogue about this casting. The hacked e-mails revealed that a Sony executive's response to the suggestion that Elba be cast was that they could not cast a black James Bond because they were concerned that the film would not be distributed internationally if they did. Casting, then, is a creative choice that has tremendous financial, social, and cognitive stakes. How do we decide what makes a trait essential to a character? When is a casting choice that runs counter to that perceived essentialism controversial and when is it celebrated for being novel or not even noticed? Though Limbaugh was being inflammatory and ridiculous on purpose, his fictive casting of Obama, Mandela, and Sharpton is not *just* wrong. It is not just that he chose three white men to play three black men; he chose actors who bring to our understanding of their portrayal of the political figures something else that Limbaugh would like to convey. Clooney's Obama would not just be white; he would also be suave and slippery. Grammer's Mandela would not highlight Mandela's actual suffering; it would convey the "perceived" suffering of Grammar's Frasier. Reiner's Sharpton would pull the teeth out of Sharpton's racial anger and replace it with a funny, Jewish irritation. Limbaugh, in just a few minutes of airtime, staged a critique of political figures through re-casting them. While Limbaugh acknowledged that Obama is real and Bond is fictional, his casting choice clarifies how large a role casting plays in our conception of the character—whether fictional or actual. The operational distinction between characters real and fictional begins to break down when both are understood as relying on, or being impacted by, conceptual casting.

Building Character draws upon research in the cognitive sciences to understand how we create character. Character is a way of organizing into memorable units the large amount of stimuli the many human beings we come into contact with provide: "my doctor," "Bond," "the president." What we do when we engage with each other—getting to know the people who play roles in our lives—is the same creative cognitive process that understands Sean Connery as a great James Bond and Rob Reiner as a disastrous Al Sharpton. This phenomenon is not magic or too beyond the fog of art to be understood from a scientific standpoint. The stakes involved in understanding this process are high, whether it is who to cast as the new Bond or how we see some public figures as likely to run for office and others as likely to cause us harm; yet the bulk of the work in this area focuses on cases where casting exposes the previous expectations about realism or mimesis. As Angela Pao points out, casting a black body in an Ibsen play has raised controversy and cries about a lack of realism when no one seems to notice that they are speaking English in Norway: "The protocols of viewing associated with translated plays are in fact so readily accepted that they provide an ironic contrast when objections to color-blind casting are made on the grounds of lack of realism."[5] Language about casting generally centers on ideas of believability or what is "right for the part," as if what the "part" called for was self-evident. When NPR reporter Wade Goodwyn wanted to convey that candidate Rick Perry—complete with new eyeglasses—looked right to run for president, he said "with his black frames and rugged good looks, Rick Perry is straight out of central casting."[6] In her important book on black performance, Brandi Wilkins Catanese calls for transgression rather than transcendence; she sees the power of expanding categories through visible casting choices, ones that evoke conversations, even if we fear the "bad manners" that may be required to talk about race and representation.[7]

Gathered into my net for analysis are actors who do not stop being themselves on film (Robert Downey Jr.) and actors who "disappear" into their characters (e.g., Daniel Day-Lewis, Meryl Streep), public figures whose performance of their role is often understood in light of the body they bring to the part (e.g., Barack Obama, Hillary Clinton), and performance conditions that can either highlight or hide the casting choice (animated films, movie trailers, presidential debates). The cognitive sciences allow us to make sense of the process; they help explain our instincts for why a particular actor is so right for a role or why race or gender matters in some political scenarios but less so in others. The process by which we build a character from the inputs of context, memory, text, and the physical properties of the body playing that character is far more powerful than has been acknowledged. Further, what is rendered visible in theatrical settings is a process we rely on but do not notice: turning the people around us into characters.

What Do I Mean by Character?

To call someone a character is not necessarily a compliment; it suggests a distinction of personality, an oversized impact, or perhaps oddity. Character actors are actors who are not cast as the leading man or woman but instead play the funny neighbor or the idiosyncratic villain. A character is also a mark on a surface or, as it was used figuratively in the fourteenth century, "the indelible quality which baptism, confirmation, and holy orders imprint on the soul."[8] The term did not refer to a person or a role until the seventeenth century. In *Character's Theater*, Lisa Freeman argues that the drama of the eighteenth century helped create a genre focused on the portrayal and circulation of identities onstage: "the eighteenth-century stage looked to the conventions of genre to provide a framework within which to measure, assess, and assign meaning to the characters represented."[9] It was this, she argued, that helped establish characters associated with individual actors who had particular kinds of value. She suggests that

> audience members did not attend Garrick's performances to see *Hamlet*, but rather to see Garrick as Hamlet. The point of eighteenth-century dramatic representations was not for the actor to transcend character, nor the character the actor, but rather for

each to be constituted in performance as visible planes of "character" that competed with and against one another for control over meaning.[10]

In the eighteenth century, then, actors did not become characters. Instead, they had "lines of business" that they were expected to portray, and if they failed to do their "part" they were "out of line."[11] This was not defined by physical characteristics as it is today; Freeman reminds us of Anne Oldfield, who "played Marcia, the virgin daughter of Cato, while she was nine months pregnant,"[12] and theater history students love to hear of actors who played ingénues into their senior years.

In the twentieth century, characters became things in themselves. Bert O. States's article "The Anatomy of Dramatic Character" seems to suggest that they can be anatomized.[13] He breaks characters into the components of Character, Personality, and Identity. Character is what results when the character confronts the events of the plot, Personality refers to baseline qualities that a character brings to the situations, and Identity is what holds these elements together in a unique manifestation at a particular time and place.[14] States's attention to the powerful entity of dramatic character is insightful, particularly as he articulated his views in *Hamlet and the Concept of Character*. For States,

> Our curiosity about character, then, is deeply centered in our need to assign more or less permanent features in a world driven by mutability and vicissitude. Before an act can be put to rest in the scheme of causality—and what interests us more than causality?— we must assign to the doer, even if the doer is nature itself, a character or quality of comportment in which we detect a certain ontological dependability.[15]

This dependability is what allows us to make sense of a narrative: we make predictions about the plot based on an assumption that a character will remain constant. Constancy operates as a stable variable in a fictional operation. In other words, each particular character "consumes experience in a special way;"[16] while the narrative may surprise us, the character is that which remains to be anatomized. Yet the metaphor of the "anatomy" in States's article presumes a body that can be isolated and extracted from its fictional and theatrical context and studied as a consistent thing; the metaphor of anatomy moves the focus of his attention to something that exists outside the perceiver, to the act of perceiving itself.

In a reading that draws upon the cognitive sciences, Blakey Vermeule takes up States's offhand quip "and what interests us more than causality?" to answer the question of the title of her book: *Why Do We Care about Literary Characters?* She points to our tendency to animate inanimate objects, as a basic human quality that is necessary for thinking about causality. Vermeule points to "conceptual primitives" that guide our construction of literary character: animism, personation, and distinguishing between the body and soul.[17] Animism refers to how we attribute life to nonliving things: "in the night, imagining some fear, / How easy is a bush supposed a bear" (*Midsummer*, 5.1.22). Personation is the automatic way we perceive others as having mental lives; persons, for Vermeule and others, are always embedded in a social situation, a narrative. Our natural tendency to separate the body and the soul allows us to see the soul as the animating part of the person and the body as the repository. Vermeule argues that literature is a place for ethical practice, where we develop a "Machiavellian intelligence" through reading the minds of characters.

Lisa Zunshine also sees our theory of mind—our ability to understand that others may have beliefs, feelings, perspectives, thoughts that are different from ours—as central to the pleasure we achieve in reading fiction.[18] In order to understand the statement "John thinks that Robert believes Jane likes him," the reader needs to be able to embed Robert's mental state ("Jane likes me") into a representation of John's mental state ("Robert believes"). Further embedded in the sentence is the evocation of Jane's mental state. Zunshine refers to this as "serially embedded representations of mental states."[19] She points to research that shows there are only so many mental states we can keep track of in order to stay in our "zone of comfort," noting that in *Mrs. Dalloway*, Virginia Woolf pushes us to hold in consciousness many different levels of intentionality. Zunshine finds in Woolf's long sentences, which traverse the perspectives of many characters, a marriage of form and function. The discomfort the reader experiences when reading these sentences provides flashes of the modern experience: there is more to see than we are capable of processing comfortably.[20]

Character, as I'm using it here and as we think of it today, is new. In Shakespeare's language, character almost exclusively referred to handwriting, or one's mark. Even when talking about how his son's behavior in Paris might impact his reputation, Polonius uses "character" to refer to the process by which the father's advice was branded into his son's memory: "And these few precepts in thy memory / Look thou character" (1.3.58–59). The idea of something "building character" dates only from the nineteenth century and was first used to refer to what happened in school classrooms.[21] Presumably, a character one "builds" in the cauldron of experiences announces integrity and proves one's worth. One Urban Dictionary user defined a "character building experience" as "any personal happening that is so absolutely awful, embarrassing, or painful that, in order to make one feel better about it, its very existence must be given some sort of arbitrary purpose, such as 'building character.'"[22] This kind of "character" relates back to the value, or "mark," engraved upon coins: it is something one can add to through experience. There are "shady" characters and people of great character. To refer to a "character" in daily life or in fiction is to integrate narrative (a presumption of past and future action) into a perception of another person.

Casting "It"

The job of the casting director is to match the actor with the character. As Richard Hicks, president of the Casting Society of

America, has said, "Finding the right actors is what makes the movie go."[23] Reading books on casting, however, will not get you any closer to understanding what makes one actor "right" and another one "wrong," nor will it give you insight into how to evaluate the character on the page for salient features to match with an actor. Books on casting, which are often aimed at actors who are trying to figure out how to get hired, provide wonderful behind-the-scenes stories of great auditions or terrible audition gaffes. They may describe the process of casting, clarifying just how much work (plus instinct and magic) goes into finding the right person for the role, but they do not say what makes one actor more right than another. While there are many books on good acting, they can't explain how a "good" actor can be bad in a particular role or how a "bad" actor can be right in a different role. Similarly, there are wonderful books on the study of character, but most of them assume that a character is a fictional, disembodied entity that preexists and outlasts the body that gives it corporeality. The rise of celebrity studies in the last thirty years suggests a powerful interest in actors who achieve renown, who seem to circulate and control our attention. Again, though, it is unclear how character, actor, and celebrity work together. Using an anecdote from a Hollywood casting office, I will briefly pull in the threads from the scholarship on celebrity, character, and casting to make clear how the three cannot be understood separately.

Rob Kendt's book on casting, *How They Cast It: An Insider's Look at Film and Television Casting*, begins with the "breakdown services," the group within a casting agency that reads the script and creates the character "breakdowns," or outlines or sketches of each character. These breakdowns are circulated to agents so they can match their clients with appropriate auditions. For example, the character of Toby Ziegler on *The West Wing* was described like this.

> In his 40s, a rumpled and sleepless Communications Director at the
> White House, Toby is Sam's boss and he works closely on a day-to-

day basis with Leo, Sam, and C. J. A man with a cynical sense of humor, Toby worries about the political implications of every decision, and is peeved with Josh for his uncalled-for remarks on *Meet the Press*. After raking Josh over the coals for having vastly exceeded the parameters of his instructions, Toby tries to preserve Josh's job by arranging a peace meeting. But when Toby attends the pow-wow with Mary Marsh and Reverend Caldwell, he blows his stack when he thinks Mary is making anti-Semitic cracks about Josh himself.[24]

Based on this breakdown, a casting director might decide that the actor needs to have the following essential qualities: an approximate age, intelligence, sense of humor, and a sense of tension or stress. The character seems written to be Jewish, but whether that is an essential qualification of the actor is open to question. The work of breakdown services is to capture in a short blurb the essential traits of the character.

Toby Ziegler is a concept made manifest in casting. According to John Levey, the casting director for *The West Wing*, two actors came through the process as strong contenders for the role of Toby: Eugene Levy and Richard Schiff. Schiff did "an outstanding reading" and "fit the Breakdown's description." Levey said, "I'd say that in all the years I've been casting, Eugene's reading was the best reading of someone who didn't get the job."[25] It is hard to imagine Levy before *American Pie*; it is hard to know if his time on *SCTV* and in *Waiting for Guffman*, combined with his eyebrows, would have been enough to make it hard to see him as a White House thinker. Levey says only that Schiff got the job because they knew his work well (from *ER*) and "we felt that there would be wider palette to draw on in the long run."[26] This certainly seems prescient, but it is unclear to me where that "palette" comes from. Is that a quality of the actor or our perception of the actor playing a character?

Perhaps Levey's analysis about the wider possible palette of Schiff came about in retrospect, after *American Pie* made it difficult to see Levy's strong eyebrows and not think of his expression when he finds his son with the apple pie in the kitchen.

As Marvin Carlson has argued, each performance is ghosted by what has come before and "each new appearance requires a renegotiation with those memories."[27] For the audience of *The West Wing*, which premiered in the same year as *American Pie* (1999), it might be challenging to renegotiate Levy-as-Jim's dad as Levy-as-White-House-communications-director-Toby Ziegler. Levy in that role might create an example of bad ghosting: as Ziegler attempted to make one of his impassioned speeches about some political issue, the audience might begin to chuckle, imagining the comic situation of the past movie in the current drama. Drawing upon the history of commedia dell'arte, Shakespeare, lines of business, and typecasting, actors have used the buildup of prior roles to their advantage. Tiffany Stern suggests that certain Shakespearean characters bear the marking of the actor who originated the role, comparing the clown roles written for Robert Armin with those written for Will Kempe: "actors may have had a series of composite character types built up over years of performance which affected every play they were in by every author."[28] According to Carlson, "The recycled body of an actor, already a complex bearer of semiotic messages, will almost inevitably in a new role evoke the ghost or ghosts of previous roles if they have made any impression whatsoever on the audience, a phenomenon that often colors and indeed may dominate the reception process."[29] Carlson explains that this ghosting works as a "reception shortcut" wherein the celebrity offers the audience an "orientation aide" to the complicated plot.[30] If these bodies are always recycled—and indeed they must be because they are not mannequins made for each performance—how is their body not marked by what has come before? Carlson seems to put the actor in a double bind here: if they have somehow failed to leave an impression on the audience in past roles, it does not speak well of their performance, but it leaves open the possibility that this past will not "color" or "dominate the reception process."[31]

There is no Oscar for best casting—the assumption seems to be that there is a simple matching procedure: connect the description in the text to the description of the actor. People point to "types" and "talent" as what is central to a casting decision, not creativity or vision. Types and talent, of course, are hard to explain or articulate. Perhaps one of the reasons casting directors have not received the creative credit they deserve is the assumption that there is a character that precedes the actor who will embody it.[32]

The tale of two Toby Zieglers—Schiff's Ziegler and Levy's Ziegler—is unfairly skewed, of course, since one Ziegler is hypothetical and the other is actual. But what if we thought about two hypothetical Ziegler's: Levy's Ziegler and Woody Allen's Ziegler? One hypothetical performance would be ghosted by a prior character while the other would be ghosted by a celebrity persona. There is a difference between an actor who has made an impact and an actor who has attained celebrity status. The influence of celebrity on a performance is not always positive. Michael Quinn's semiotic reading of casting says that although there is "something about dramatic performance that causes spectators to seek information about the personal life of the performer," celebrities intrude in the "creative genius" of the author or director.[33] And yet nobody sells tickets like a celebrity.

The body of the actor and his/her history is always onstage with the character. Familiarity is a positive element of a production in most cases. We are used to conflating the actor's body and the character's body so that when Meryl Streep is playing Margaret Thatcher or Daniel Day-Lewis is playing Lincoln, our attention is drawn to the virtuoso of the mimesis. The fact that Streep is not British or Day-Lewis is not American drops away. But when Idris Elba is to play Bond or Helen Mirren is to play Prospero, we are suddenly aware of bodies. Some bodies pass more seamlessly than others. It is not easy to separate questions of charisma and celebrity, or what Joseph Roach would call "It," from the dynamic interplay of casting and character.[34]

While there is tremendous interest in questions of charisma and celebrity and some work has been done on the phenomenology of fictional characters, the topic of casting, of fitting the celebrity to the role, is undertheorized. Moreover, the brilliant scholars working on celebrity rarely engage with the brilliant scholars writing about character. Although at first glance they are separate areas, I argue that they are inseparable. Roach has exploded notions of performance in his work, examining "how culture reproduces and re-creates itself by a process that can be best described by the word *surrogation*."[35] The memory carries forward through substitution; Lady Gaga is not Britney Spears is not Madonna is not Marilyn Monroe, but these "effigies," "provide communities with a method of perpetuating themselves through specially nominated mediums or surrogates: among them, actors, dancers, priests, street maskers, statesmen, celebrities, freaks, children, and especially, by virtue of an intense but surprising paradox, corpses."[36]

In his theorizing of the role of actor as effigy, Roach quotes George Farquhar speaking about a performance of Thomas Betterton: "'Yet the whole Audience at the same time knows that this is Mr. Betterton, who is strutting upon the Stage, and tearing his Lungs for a Livelihood. And that the same Person shou'd be Mr. Betterton, and Alexander the Great, at the same Time, is somewhat like an Impossibility, in my Mind.'"[37] Audiences held these multiple understandings simultaneously—Betterton is an actor strutting on a stage and Betterton is Alexander the Great—to form a constellation of things that define what is being watched. What Farquhar finds to be "somewhat like an Impossibility" is the same cognitive ability that children use to understand a banana as a phone or a doll as a baby. Isolating something as one thing instead of an amorphous assemblage of potentials is a far more complicated cognitive task. In the same way that we can come to understand the place where several streets come together as an "intersection"—an identity that is dependent on but encompasses the constituent parts—we can understand disparate, complicated stimuli as a "character."

My goal here is to explore the cognitive process that takes place at the intersection of stimuli—what is salient, what disappears—when a body struts and frets in front of us and a character is born. How do we calibrate performances so we can manage the associations that a character evokes in order to make sense of him or her? In other words, how do we attend to some information and not others? For Carlson, the stage is haunted by many ghosts—the space, the text, and the bodies—and while I do not disagree with him, I want to know where the ghosting stops. In other words, because all cognition is haunted by memories and directed by expectations, I am interested in how we reduce the number of "ghosts." How do we simplify the stimuli so they are manageable and even enjoyable? When Meryl Streep was cast as Margaret Thatcher, she had already played many powerful parts. In addition, Margaret Thatcher was a real person. Thus, people brought to the film associations and expectations about both Streep and Thatcher.[38] Yet critics and audience members seemed to be able to follow Streep as Thatcher. We were affected by Streep's performance without being confused by all the other characters Streep has played. Some ghosts didn't show up.

In the special issue of *PMLA* on "Celebrity, Fame, Notoriety," editors Joseph A. Boone and Nancy J. Vickers began their introduction by discussing fame as something more powerful than character or talent: "That Susan Boyle had millions of fans around the world within twenty-four hours or that Barack Obama 'arguably won the presidency because of his effectiveness at mobilizing [traditional and Internet] media spectacle' powerfully attests to the fact that we have entered a new era that demands new tools of analysis."[39] Some of the tools we should mobilize in understanding character, talent, performance, and the reception process come from the cognitive sciences. If the reception process can be so deeply affected by the dynamics of celebrity, timing, history, context, race, and gender, then we need to question how we understand this "reception process." It must not be strictly semiotic or computational; a computer trained to assess talent and star-potential would not have predicted Susan Boyle's impact. We do not "read" people in a static, hermetically sealed environment. What I want to propose here is a cognitive approach to theatrical character and a theatrical understanding of a central component of cognition—categorization—as casting.

Casting is historically and temporally contingent. Our under-standing of a character, like all cognition, happens in the flow of time, based on memories, predictions, and anticipations. We return to past assumptions with new information and reinter-pret and remember. Roger Moore's Bond fit his age just as Daniel Craig's Bond fit his. While Eugene Levy might have been a ter-rific Toby Ziegler before *American Pie*, a Toby Ziegler ghosted by Jim's dad would not have had the gravitas needed for the White House. Cognition depends on the taking and changing of view-points, and our comprehension of character, of casting, depends on where and when we stand. Instead of "reading" a particular performance or work of art, which necessarily pulls it out of its context and out of the flow of time, I want to take a theatrical point of view, to understand the building of characters as dy-namic, embedded, and creative.

We use the metaphor "read" when we say what an object or a text means to us. In this metaphor, when we read an object, a text, a play, or a situation, we take in information linearly and turn it into an interpretation. Our disembodied eye takes in a string of words and enters them into the processing system in the brain, which generates an interpretation. While this is a pow-erful metaphor for meaning-making, it omits key elements of the experience of reading, let alone performance. I do not think we read linearly or semiotically and we certainly don't take in performances this way. Traditionally, we have taken the herme-neutic moment out of time, thinking about meaning as some-thing stable and out there in the environment to be taken into our heads and processed. What do I mean by meaning? Meaning can suggest a mental precept or belief in correlation with some-thing external to the self. The fact that my feet are wet *means* that I have just stepped into the water. I want to add honey to my cereal and this *means* that I want it sweeter. "I eat you up I love you so" *means* that my love for you is like a hunger—I desire to take you in and make you a part of me. Two plus two *means* four. The last sentence has been generally thought of as the least figurative, the most literal, with "means" here being more like "equal to." Yet work by George Lakoff and Rafael Núñez suggests that our experience with addition is just as metaphoric at its root as our experience with literature: both begin and end with embodied engagement with the world.[40] Meaning is a dynamic process of connection. Lakoff and Mark Johnson argue (with others) that the "body and brain are where meanings arise in and through our interactions with the environment and other people."[41] The plural form of meaning may be what can be most useful; just as there are multiple meanings of "now is the winter of discontent," there are multiple meanings of "honey" and "wet feet."

Casting a Net: Binding, Categories, and Cognition

Cognitive science provides new tools for reimagining the "reception process" that makes Sean Connery or Idris Elba James Bond. To say that cognition is embodied means more than that the brain is part of the body and thus impossible to fully separate from it. It means more than the fact the brain isn't a computer operating "off site" and then sending messages to the body. It means that thinking is what happens when I am in my body. It means that imagining an eagle and seeing an eagle use many of the same cells. Subjects shown a picture of a flying eagle after reading the sentence "The ranger saw an eagle in the sky," far more quickly identified the image as matching a word mentioned in the sentence then when they were shown an image of an eagle perched on a tree.[42] As Benjamin Bergen summarizes: "It appears quite natural for people understanding language to produce embodied simulations of the things that they read or hear about."[43] Embodied cognition means that the meaning carried by the shape our mouths take in saying a word is part of our experience of that word. In one experiment, given the choice between associating an unknown word with a spiky object or a curved object, 95 percent of the study participants associated "kiki" with a spiky object and "bouba" with a curved object. The researchers hypothesized that the shape the participants' mouths made as they said the words guided their associations.[44]

The first generation of cognitive science did imagine the brain as a computer, and that model defined how they thought about thinking and the experiments they did. The "embodiment prem ise," as Raymond Gibbs defines it, on the other hand, imagines a different set of assumptions from which to design experiments. According to Gibbs,

> People's subjective felt experiences of their bodies in action pro-
> vide part of the fundamental grounding for language and thought.
> Cognition is what occurs when the body engages the physical, cul-
> tural world and must be studied in terms of the dynamical interac-
> tions between people and the environment. Human language and
> thought emerge from recurring patterns of embodied activity that
> constrain ongoing intelligent behavior. We must not assume cog-
> nition to be purely internal, symbolic, computational, and disem-
> bodied, but seek out the gross and detailed ways that language and
> thought are inextricably shaped by embodied action.[45]

While this book will not explore all the implications of Gibbs's premise for theater scholarship, it takes it as the basis for asking and answering questions about our engagement with characters and actors.[46]

A growing body of research suggests that comprehending language is a full-bodied affair. Although there is still some debate in the sciences about the relationships among language, cognition, the body, and consciousness, studies suggest that we do not have an isolated language section of the brain that takes conscious experience as input and returns words as output. Factors such as the condition of the body can also influence interpretation. The state of the body is not just an input in language interpreta tion; it is also an output. For example, in one study, researchers learned that when participants read the words "she handed me back the letter," they were much quicker to perform the action of moving their hands toward their bodies than the action of moving their hands away from their bodies, suggesting that comprehension of the sentence accesses the motor cortex sufficiently to prime one physical action (movement toward) over another (movement away).[47] Others have extended this kind of result to show that the hand muscles are primed even by sentences that describe metaphorical exchanges ("You delegate the responsibilities to Anna.").[48]

A critical early moment in the history of embodied cognition came in 1954, when J. J. Gibson and his wife E. J. Gibson argued against the behaviorist psychology that prevailed at the time and for an ecological approach to perception and learning. For the Gibsons, the agent making sense of her environment does so relative to herself. If she is making piecrust, the rolling pin is a tool to flatten the dough; if she is defending her life, the rolling pin becomes a weapon. The rolling pin gains its meaning when it is used for one thing rather than another, prior to that it is potential. Tables function differently for humans and for dogs and thus they mean different things to humans and dogs. This may seem obvious, but the key point is that humans interact with their world in much the same way a dog does: what elements of our environment are good for sitting and which are good for climbing and which are good for resting? Although language complicates how we represent our world, we are still capable of coming across a strange object and seeing it as something that accommodates sitting, even if it isn't a chair.

How we speak of that chair, of a table, or of a mountain in the distance comes from our experience of interacting with the world physically. The conceptual metaphor theory of George Lakoff, Mark Johnson, and Mark Turner argues that we borrow or make use of information about our experience in our bodies to makes sense of more abstract concepts. We understand the abstract in terms of the concrete and physical.[49] When we say that a theory is getting clearer, it is not just that we are making metaphoric the process of comprehension, it is that we think about thinking as a process of seeing; we think metaphorically. We say

"I see what you mean" not because we see anything, but because we understand knowledge through connection to our visual system. This connection between domains or experiences, allows us to borrow, or in their terms, project, information from one domain onto our experience with another. I can project my experience pouring water into a container where the more water I pour, the higher it goes to understand the stock market going up or receiving a high salary. The warmth of my mother's embrace structures my experience of love and kindness later in life, so that we can speak of being in a warm relationship or about a person who seems cold. We think and speak metaphorically.

Gilles Fauconnier and Mark Turner have shown that some things are not metaphors; instead, they are an integration network of two or more concepts or "mental spaces."[50] Conceptual integration theory (or blending) suggests that we use compression in all of our thinking and speaking as a way of connecting networks of associations, from the concrete and the physical to the abstract or the theoretical. Compression is the process whereby something diffuse and large—like a dynamic weather system—can be reduced to something smaller and simpler—like a map with swirling colors on it. Once something is compressed, we can project information accessed from that mental space— color means temperature, movement means change over time, that map shows where I live—to an understanding of what the weather will be tomorrow. We do not project all the information from the picture—we don't think the rain will suddenly be the color green. Integration theory argues that we make meaning through this creative networking: the connection between two or more mental spaces generates emergent properties that are not present in the original, separate input spaces. This is not a combination or a blurring of two ideas, it is a complicated network that we evoke and integrate to create a new idea. This is how, as I hope to show, the body of Idris Elba, the character of James Bond, and the history of race relations in America can come together to create a character so vibrant and disturbing as to occupy the time of Rush Limbaugh.

Integration theory builds on Fauconnier's theory of mental spaces, which he defines as "constructs distinct from linguistic structures but built up in any discourse according to guidelines provided by the linguistic expressions."[51] These are packets of information in which humans organize information that we construct and frame on the fly. Mental space theory provides a model for a process of constructing meaning that is fluid and expandable, capable of explaining examples in language that the more complicated logical theories cannot, such as "If I were you, I'd hate me," co-reference, and propositional problems.[52] Some words are prompts for meaning; these are "space builders," such as "Max believes" or "In that movie" that set up a space that informs and/or structures the words/information to come.[53] "Max believes Sarah went to the store," for example, creates an event that is understood in relation to what Max believes. These spaces are not unlike the "domains" Lakoff referred to as "target" and "source" or to or what is implied by the "tenor" and "vehicle" designations of I. A. Richards's understanding of metaphors.[54] In *The Way We Think*, Fauconnier and Turner argue that these spaces come together in meaning composition in networks. This process is not complex, weird, advanced, or literary; it is routine and omnipresent.

Perhaps the best example of an integration network for our purposes is the "Bypass" advertisement that Fauconnier and Turner present. In the picture, there are three kids dressed in surgical gear, a body on the table in front of them and scalpels in their hands, staring at the camera. The headline below them reads: "Joey, Katie, and Todd will be performing your bypass."[55] The threatening scenario of children performing heart bypass surgery is intended to persuade the viewer to read the text in the body of the ad, which explains that our education system is not training our students in the kinds of skills and knowledge they will need to be good doctors in the future. If you thought that the reduction of standards in America's education system would not affect you, the scenario vividly dramatizes exactly the moment you will wish you supported education. As Fauconnier explains:

Joey, Katie, and Todd in one space are children yet to be educat-
ed. In the other input space, they are doctors whose formal education lies behind them. The cross-space mapping connects the child
to the adult. Both are projected to the blend, partially, and fused
there. We also project to the blend the frame of surgery that comes
from the space with the adults. The surgeons in the blend are seven-
year-olds, which is naturally terrifying. We want our surgeons to
be more competent than seven-year-olds, which leads us directly to
the question of how to turn the children into competent adults.[56]

The ad requires us to compress and connect the concepts of children, doctors, students, adults, now, and the future. We don't
actually think that in the future seven-year-olds will be allowed
to perform surgery; we compress the concept of the intellect and
skill of the kids with the role of the doctor. There is also a cause-
and-effect link between now and then: the effect of bad doctors
in the future comes from the cause of poor education now. Notice
that this is information made manifest in the blend, but it is not
at all direct. Spending money on education does not guarantee
that your bypass will be a success. Educating these three children
won't guarantee it either. In the network staged in this ad, however, the effect of not spending on education leads directly to the
effect: your terribly scary surgery. As Fauconnier explains, "The
emergent meaning in the blend in this case includes fear and anxiety, which are not necessarily attached to the inputs."[57] Casting
the doctors in this way creates an emergent meaning that does
not come from the "parts" (surgeons) or from the "script" ("Joey,
Katie, and Todd will be performing your bypass"); it comes from
the blend created by the casting.[58] Understanding that "casting"
is the process by which we generate an integration network from
character (surgeon) and actor (seven-year-old) complicates and
extends Fauconnier and Turner's argument.

In *The Way We Think*, Fauconnier and Turner refer to the conceptual blend that is created when an actor takes the stage:

> The character portrayed may of course be entirely fictional, but
> there is still a space, a fictional one, in which that person is alive.

We do not go to a performance of *Hamlet* in order to measure the similarity between the actor and a historical prince of Denmark. The power comes from the integration in the blend. The spectator is able to live in the blend, looking directly on its reality. . . . The importance and power of living in the blend would be hard to overestimate.[59]

Embodied by the actor, "Hamlet" can become Hamlet and "Bond" can become Bond. The actor is never invisible, never wholly subsumed by the identity of the character: "While we perceive a single scene, we are simultaneously aware of the actor moving and talking on a stage in front of an audience, and of the corresponding character moving and talking within the represented story world."[60] Fauconnier and Turner are correct to perceive that the audience is neither in a trance state nor "suspending disbelief"[61] but I would like to complicate the idea of "living in the blend" that Bruce McConachie and I have picked up. McConachie applies this to an understanding of actor/character as "a blend of real people and fictional people whom audiences readily credit with real intentions and emotions when they live in the blend while watching a play."[62] McConachie and I have referred to this character/actor blend with a slash, but I worry that this oversimplifies the complicated network. As Turner says, "A blend is not a small abstraction of the mental spaces it blends and it is not a partial cut-and-paste assembly, either, because it contains new stuff, new ideas. It is a tight, packed little compression. It contains much less information than the full mental web it serves. From it, we can reach up to manage and work on the rest of the vast mental web."[63] Conceptual integration networks offer a model for thinking about character onstage (and thus about casting decisions) in terms of a dynamic multiplicity of spaces and information.

Since Plato and Aristotle, we have been thinking about the relationship between the "original" and the representation. As I have discussed elsewhere, the Chorus in *Henry V* shares this worry, starting the play with an articulation of the representation failure of what's to come:

O for a Muse of fire, that would ascend
The brightest heaven of invention,
A kingdom for a stage, princes to act
And monarchs to behold the swelling scene!
Then should the warlike Harry, like himself,
Assume the port of Mars, and at his heels
(Leash'd in, like hounds) should famine, sword, and fire
Crouch for employment. (0.2–9)

The fictional play will, he insists, be continually haunted by the reality of the historical truth. This is a narrator who announces at the start that "you should have been there," since to do justice to this history, there should be no substitution or representation: the part of King Henry should be played by King Henry. The Chorus wants us to imagine a blend of now and then, history and fiction, where the warlike Harry and the actor are one, where monarchs behold monarchs.

The spinning of a counterfactual tale is what sets the stage for the particular blend I want to focus on here. In the "like himself" conceptual network, the king is able to replace the king because they are related through analogy, but one is dead and the other needs to be alive. The historical king was never singular either, since he was a decidedly *unwarlike* youth in the *Henry IV* plays and it was only at the end of *Henry V* that one would consider him "warlike." (Indeed, when the play begins, the dauphin of France is so convinced that Henry would never be "warlike" that he mocks the new king by sending him tennis balls.) The one man who will play the part of King Henry will be *made up* of the historical King Henry—the one at the end of the story we are about to hear, not the one at the beginning, where the character must begin.[64] Shakespeare's language and theatrical conventions of representation call our attention to the ways we make up characters at the site of intersecting stimuli. Audiences need to link a complicated network of spaces to replace the role with the man, to make one (King Henry) equal one (this King Henry). The Chorus makes visible the casting of an actor who will play this character and the casting that turned the "original" King Henry into a "warlike king." The "warlike king" was also always already a fictional character created at the intersection of a network; Shakespeare stages a new network while the Chorus points out the work done in creating both.

I turn toward blending theory and other research in cognitive science because it helps me ask and answer questions critical within my discipline. I am not interested in being a disciplinary tourist; I am interested in being a disciplinary ambassador. I want cognitive scientists to understand and address the questions we are asking and answering in the humanities, and I want scholars in the humanities to explore and probe the research being done in the sciences. Because those who work in cognitive linguistics and those who work in literary studies both aim to understand language in a rich and embedded way, this makes combining the two fields particularly fruitful for dialogue. F. Elizabeth Hart boldly claims that blending theory will

> be the aspect of cognitive linguistics that has the most lasting impact on literary studies, and here, in brief, is why: theirs is a theory of meaning that acknowledges the postmodern problematics of interpretation (the view of where we've been) while at the same time addressing our need to comprehend the mechanics of even imperfect meaning and interpretation (the view of where we'd like to go).[65]

She is speaking to both the dead end of poststructuralist conceptions of language and the incredible importance of contingency in meaning. Conceptual blending theory can expose the conceptual structures that keep problematic narratives and paradigms in place and offer a tremendous tool to those of us who want to know how and why stories are told by bodies onstage. Several important works have integrated blending theory into literary studies, but few have examined its impact on theater scholarship.[66] An application of blending theory to theater and performance confronts the complexity of a meaning-making event that includes the bodies of the participants, unlike literature, for example, where the character's body is constructed from words.[67]

How we categorize, how we conceive of the world around us, impacts what we are capable of seeing, what we are capable of knowing. Teaching babies to talk is teaching them to categorize: "Where's the doggy? What sound does the doggy make? Where's the blue ball?" As we teach babies to label, we are teaching them to categorize based on the distinctions that are most important in our culture. In most romance languages, the world is categorized by gender; you cannot say "la chien" because "dog" is masculine. In some languages, how you know something (I heard or know indirectly versus I saw it first hand) is encoded into verb tense. Some languages give all directions based on absolute coordinates: "to get to the school, go 500 paces NW, then 300 paces E." Some languages encode the world around them based on elements of the local landscape. "In Guugu Yimithirr, rather than asking someone to 'move back from the table,' one might say, 'move a bit to the mountain.'"[68] Because how we speak is how we think, cognitive linguistics has played an important role in exposing how we make sense out of the endless stimuli that flows our way.

I cannot calculate pi to the tenth place or tell you how many times in the last ten pages I have typed the word "the." Although a computer can do those tasks very well, it cannot recognize the coffee cup in front of me. This is called the "binding" or "grounding" problem—"how the symbols are mapped back onto the real world"—and it has been an incredibly generative problem in cognitive sciences.[69] If computers can't compute how to tell the difference between the mug and the background, perhaps we have mistakenly assumed that thinking was computing. Certain features of the environment are processed in specific locations of the brain. For example, within the visual system, the cones process color and the rods process light. The binding problem is understanding how these features, which are processed in distinct brain regions, come back together again to give us a whole.

There are actually seven types of binding. In "property binding," the color, say, of the ball must be bound to the ball. In "part binding," the handle on the cup must be seen as part of the cup and not as the background. In location binding, the "what" of an object (a mug) must be bound to the "where" of it (on the desk). Because of a stroke or a particular form of brain damage, some people have apperceptive agnosia and cannot recognize objects in their environment. They can see perfectly well, but they cannot easily perceive the seemingly obvious unity of the mug as different from the desk. The loss of this ability in some is evidence that it is an ability the rest of us have. Just as we can distinguish the coffee cup from the desk, we can distinguish the man behind the counter from the man holding our hand.[70] This is the cognitive work that brings the figure forward from the ground—whether it is a hammer, a coffee cup, or a face—and gives it unity.[71] Once there are all these figures, of course, we need a system for categorizing them. Before there is a character, an actor, or a spectator, there must be a cognitive system that is capable of organizing stimuli into these categories. Imagine trying to understand James Bond if you couldn't keep Bond separate from M or M separate from Felix Leiter.

Imagine a creature with a similar physical makeup to yourself—one with legs, arms, torso, eyes, etc.—who does not have the ability to assign, say, "chair" to environmental objects upon which she sits. Every encounter with the environment for her would be a first time, a set of perceptions that affords actions—pull hand away from the hot thing, rest on that smooth thing.[72] Then imagine that this creature evolves a kind of cognitive lasso that she can use to group elements in her environment that afford similar actions: all these things from which I must run, all these things upon which I can rest. Now she has categories and objects in her environment, not just perceptions. As she goes along, she will add to and change her categories; instead of just a category for things to run from, she might have "large animals with teeth" and "fire," as these two categories might necessitate a slightly different flight path. The categories allow us to offload cognition; they improve our intelligence and our efficiency.

In the 1970s, Eleanor Rosch, a psychologist at the University of California, Berkeley, showed that categories are defined by prototypes, not by necessary and sufficient conditions. This means that our category of "chair" may be defined by a dining room chair but can be expanded to include a barstool or a beanbag. Categories are not objective groups; they are created as a tool. Based on years of studying color recognition in speakers of the Dani tribe in New Guinea, Rosch and her colleagues showed that although the Dani speakers did not have words for certain colors, they could see them and have a conceptual category for them; their language did not wholly determine their conceptual system. Thus, she argues, "human categorization should not be considered the arbitrary product of historical accident or of whimsy but rather the result of psychological principles of categorization, which are subject to investigation."[73] This insight suggests that we can investigate, think through, and alter our categories. Because how we categorize is so deeply enmeshed with how we think, this is a powerful idea.

George Lakoff's 1989 book *Women, Fire, and Dangerous Things* takes its title from a different way of categorizing the world. In Dyirbal, an Australian aboriginal language, all objects are classified in one of four ways, but the four classifications are not immediately obvious. For example, the first includes men and most animals, spears, and storms. The second includes women, bandicoots, most birds, the hairy mary grub, and things connected with water and fire. What Lakoff argues, extending the work of the anthropologist who conducted the fieldwork, is that the objects are grouped based on "the domain-of-experience principle: If there is a basic domain of experience associated with A, then it is natural for entities in that domain to be in the same category as A."[74] What accounts for the most striking of the aberrant cases (the hairy mary grub, for example, should be in group one since it is an insect but is in group two) is the "myth and belief principle," which privileges the myth or belief about a thing over what those outside the group would see as its "objective" taxonomy. The hairy mary grub is classified with the sun in group two because its sting feels like a sunburn. For Lakoff, the extraordinary contribution of this anthropological study is its explanation of how categories are created through experience. What from our perspective looks fantastical (grouping women, fire, and hairy mary grubs) "is from the perspective of the people doing the classifying a relatively regular and principled way to classify things."[75] What we lasso with our rope depends upon where we stand and what we need.

According to the old, "objectivist" view of cognition, categories inhered in the things themselves, on objectively assessed, shared properties. The category "dogs" referred to furry domesticated animals that bark and the category "light" referred to waves of energy. Based on many different experiments and studies in the fields of anthropology, neuroscience, linguistics, philosophy, and biology (among others), it became clear that these distinctions did not exist in the world around us—there is no hidden "canis" mark on all the animals we have placed in the category of dog. Instead, they exist in our cognitive system, which is inseparable from the bodies we have and the environment we live in. Therefore, cognition is not some disembodied process that happens in the brain: cognition is embodied. We do not just think differently because of the bodies we have, we think with and through the bodies we have. Though cognitive scientists debate about how far to take this approach, there is very little debate that categories are not based on predefined necessary and sufficient conditions; they are based on prototypes and are thus changeable.

We create categories conceptually; nowhere in our brain is there a circle labeled "mammals" that contains animals that give birth to live babies; nurse their young; have hair, three bones in the middle ear, and a neocortex; and are warm-blooded. Categories include "cognitive reference points" and "prototypes" that *organize* them but do not *define* them. The category "dog" is not an entity in the world the way "Fluffy" is. We may have a prototype for "mammal" or "doctor" that includes some animals or some people but not others. Because how we speak is how we think, these can have real-world consequences. If you do not believe that categories are created, you cannot imagine changing them. Understanding that our categories are negotiable, that we can decide whether it is more useful to categorize relationships around prototype A than around prototype B, has huge implications for how we see each other and how we live. Usually a category does not break down until the evidence against its utility is so overwhelming—say when an experiment shows evidence that light functions like a particle or when a society expands who counts as human after many years of violent political struggle—but there are always artists and scientists who are willing to see beyond the limits of current categories.

Once the research in cognitive linguistics and embodied cognition has persuaded you that our brains do not arbitrarily assign words to things out there in the world via a system of difference, that we do not process language like a code, that we do not have a Freudian subconscious, then it follows that some reconsideration of literary and performance theory is necessary. By connecting the phenomenon to theories in cognitive science, we are able to connect important work in theater and performance studies with ideas about how we experience daily life. If I can argue for the implications of research in theater and performance in a way that makes sense across the disciplines, perhaps there can be a mutually beneficial conversation. To cast a part, a casting director is underlining and creating similarities between an actor and words on the page. A theory of what this process is should take into consideration research from the cognitive sciences about perception and categorization. It should appreciate the complexity and the stakes of the issue. To cast characters is to create them, to bring them to life, and, thus, control the spectator's expectations about them. Casting is the reduction of dimensions. It is creative and transformational. Though done most visibly by casting directors, all of us create characters by connecting bodies with roles. Characters, then, are a by product of a cognitive system that can cast people. In this way, all characters are fictional.

Casting About

One of the central interests of this book is category construction: how we organize information to make it most useful to us. It is no surprise, then, that my decisions about how to divide the book into chapters suggests how I imagine readers will read this book. Of course, I trust that the reader will begin enthusiastically at the beginning and remain in the grip of my argument and prose until the last endnote, but I also recognize the need for efficiency and a narrowing of interest. While there will be an accumulation of the scientific information supporting my larger argument, I have also divided the book so that readers with particular interests can experience the book through the lens with which they are most comfortable. One could read this book by starting with the most familiar example in the index and allowing that passage to initiate a second index probe. The selection of the chapters and the order of the argument, however, is meant to lead the reader from the basic cognitive process that makes casting possible to the elements that impact that processing in practice, to some of the powerful theatrical work this process enables artists and performers to do, to some of the implications of that work for our daily lives and for our conception of the self in general.

Chapter 1, "Building Titus: Compressing the Complex into the Essential," begins by discussing trailers, celebrities, names, and faces as examples of compression. We compress what is complicated and diffuse into something that is focused and essential in order to decrease our cognitive load, increase associations, and facilitate memory. The chapter ranges widely in order to focus on compression: it begins with Heath Ledger's painted face in the trailer for *The Dark Knight* (2008) and ends with research on how we process the faces we love (such as the face of our mother) and celebrity faces (such as the face of Jennifer Aniston).

Chapter 2, "Building Characters: Seeing Bodies," examines actors who "disappear" into their characters and actors who do not. Meryl Streep can be Karen Silkwood, Margaret Thatcher, or Julia Child while Robert Downey Jr. creates Ironman Robert Downey Jr. I argue that this is not just a question of talent. I examine the impact of celebrity, the ghosts of parts past—such as in the casting of James Gandolfini as Carol in *Where the Wild Things Are*—and actors without ghosts who bring complexity to characters—such as Tatiana Maslany in *Orphan Black*. Our brains derive narrative or conceptual information from the collision between an actor's body and a character's role. This allows us to offload complex conclusions to the network of associations that are evoked when this particular body plays this particular part. Some bodies, I find, do not seem to disappear as easily as others into their parts. I analyze the performance of the same song by two different artists at different times (Dr. Dre and Ben Folds) and the same actor playing the same character after many years. The debate over casting whites to play nonwhite parts in plays such as *The Mountaintop* and the hysteria over Carrie Fisher's weight demonstrates the critical roadblocks that some actors face. Because cognition is embedded in an environment, I also talk about how we build characters in networks; the casting of Juliet, of course, depends upon the casting of Romeo.

Chapter 3, "Multicasting: The Dispersed Character," focuses on more strangely built characters found in Michelangelo's *Pietà*, the star-studded and multi-character run of Eve Ensler's *The Vagina Monologues*, and the documentary theater work of Anna Deavere Smith. This chapter aims to extend my argument about casting to argue that our comprehension of others, our building of character, is dynamic, embedded, and creative.

Chapter 4, "Casting and the Performance of Everyday Life," argues that the process we use to build characters in fiction is the process we use to categorize those around us into roles. I extend the argument to understand how we select candidates for public office and how certain events can transform our casting of others and ourselves. Rape, torture, abuse, and war can all forcibly cast a person against his/her will. Some things change everything.

Chapter 5, "Counter Casting: Building Colony" uses the concept of casting to put pressure on the idea of the self. If casting is how we come up with ideas of the others, it is also how we contain our idea of our self. I argue that the creativity involved in casting also suggests ways that we might reimagine our selves and our ecosystems.

This book is not about acting or about celebrity or popular culture, although those things will be important because they provide ways to perceive the impact of casting. It is not a book about casting Shakespeare plays, although Shakespeare remains a critical cultural touchstone and the casting of Shakespeare's plays is particularly visible and crucial given the amount of cognitive work the actors' bodies take on in communicating Shakespeare to a contemporary audience. Although there is a literature in cognitive film studies, this book will not engage with those approaches.[76] It is also not a book about the history of interesting or problematic casting choices. This book is about the seemingly seamless process of category construction, compression, and casting, processes by which we jump to powerful conclusions that it is our duty to challenge. This is a relatively short book: I am outlining an area for future research and a methodology for that exploration. It is intentionally broad in scope—I analyze casting in a rap song, a Renaissance sculpture, and a contemporary children's film—and this is critical to assessing the phenomenon underlying these disparate examples.

CHAPTER 1

BUILDING TITUS

Compressing the Complex into the Essential

When we watch a movie trailer, we understand that things are being left out. Several hours of story are reduced to quick shots, dramatic narration, and (often) loud music. They do not always work, either because they fail to seduce their target audience (as measured in ticket sales) or because they seem to misrepresent the film. The trailer for Christopher Nolan's *Dark Knight* (2008) succeeded in conveying the dark turn the franchise was taking by starting with a voice intoning over dismal shots of the city that "this city deserves a better class of criminal," adding (as the trailer cuts to Heath Ledger as the Joker) "and I'm going to give it to 'em." Though the rest of the trailer gives the standard superhero fare of explosions, fast-moving vehicles, and men in masks, Ledger's painted face returns again and again to remind the audience of the film's commitment to a truly scary and dark film.[1] Ledger may not have been an obvious choice, but the trailer quickly conveys how right he was.

Casting, like trailers, works to reduce the possibilities of a character. This takes advantage of the cognitive process of compression: the same shorthand I rely on when I see a line drawing and know it represents a face. In this chapter, I examine the shorthand that celebrity casting creates as visible in trailers. I argue that we use compression in casting, in naming, and in per-

ceiving faces to efficiently make sense of the present and anticipate the future. Scientists researching facial recognition suggest
that social navigation and the perception of characters are influ-
enced by this biological process.

Compression

Each winter, weather experts point to satellite images of the
country with swirling colors that represent frigid temperatures
and snow. When the weather man or woman points to a picture
of earth with colors moving over it, TV audiences understand
that it is not the case that the map is being assaulted by colors;
the graphic compresses the weather changes on the earth to a
flat, visual image. The winter of 2014 was particularly cold in the
U.S. Midwest. Temperatures that were normal for the polar region had come south and the Midwest experienced a polar vortex. Soon a picture of the graphic was circulating on social media
with text that said: "Go home Polar Vortex: You're drunk."[2] This
makes no sense, of course, and yet the fact that it circulated so
widely suggests that I was not the only one who found it funny.
Figuring out why it is funny reveals a cognitive process that is
not just reserved for Internet memes.

Maps are an excellent example of compression. We compress
a large and detailed physical environment to a scale that is useful for tracking weather patterns. Compression is a term for the
unconscious process by which we reduce the scale of something.
According to Fauconnier and Turner, in a network of mental
spaces, some spaces share "vital relations," such as in the bypass
ad example I discussed in the previous chapter, the concept of
cause and effect: the idea that a lack of education causes bad doctors. In that case, the time between cause and effect has been
compressed, so that the lack of education today results in a bad
surgery minutes from now. In the map example, a dynamic experience of weather over time is presented as a colorful picture in

space. As Mark Johnson reminds us, maps are not actually there: "We do not experience the *maps*, but rather *through them* we experience a structured world full of patterns and qualities."[3] We experience what the maps make it possible to perceive. Where we are in space, the relationship of our location to changing weather, our need for scarves and hats this morning, and the likelihood that our commute home this afternoon will be very difficult can be efficiently communicated by moving colors on a flat screen. The vast and complicated data that makes air cool down and travel, producing extreme changes in our environment, can be brought to a human scale by compressing the size of the country onto a four-foot screen and translating the range of weather fluctuations into color variations. The color spectrum and the range of temperatures we experience share variation by degree, so we can understand that the difference between cold and hot temperatures has been compressed through analogy to the difference between blue and red on the color spectrum. As Fauconnier and Turner explain,

> Compression is a way to achieve human scale, and by the same token achieving human scale will produce compression. . . . The compression and scale of the blend make it more tractable to deal with, more manipulable, and since it is tied to the complex network, its manipulation gives mastery of a diffuse network, which creates a feeling of global conceptual mastery and insight. Going from many elements and relations in the network to few in the blend also helps achieve human scale, compression, and stories, because a simple human-scale scenario, with a minimal number of agents in a local spatial region and a small temporal interval, is what we are set up to engage with perceptually and behaviorally.[4]

Weather maps reduce the vast spaces around us and the unpredictable changes in our experiences to a size and scale we can understand.

Once this compression is set up, the text of the Internet

meme prompts us to stage an alternate story: the weaving color lines become an entity named Polar Vortex that is behaving erratically and inappropriately because it's drunk. Although the image is actually a map of the United States, we "see" a character where none exists. A weather event has been cast as a different kind of nuisance: a lost and disorderly drunk. The drunk character evokes memories of experiences of dealing with drunk people, both the possible damage they can cause and the temporary nature of the problem: a drunk can go home, in this case back to the polar region, and sober up. The joke also casts the viewer as the stable, sober person capable of castigating a powerful force. With a few lines and colors, the image has prompted us to create two characters in a story: the lost drunk and the sober authority.

This chapter will examine how we compress what is complicated and diffuse into what is focused and essential in order to decrease cognitive load, increase associations, and facilitate memory. Characters, like categories, do not exist in the world: we create them to make sense of our perceptions. We build character through a dynamic interplay between a number of conceptual spaces: the body (age, race, gender, physical attributes); textual information (actions taken or lines said about or by the character); what we know already or anticipate based on historical information, personal information about the character, and the actor portraying it; the reputation of the character (and the actor); and what we know about other roles the actor's body has taken on. We build the Polar Vortex character by projecting the information about the colors on the map, the text that refers to the entity being drunk, our previous experience with miserable and inconvenient cold weather, and our previous experience with miserable and inconvenient drunks. These come together to make us laugh because we can play in that dynamic space: for example, by restaging yesterday's shoveling of the driveway as cleaning up after a drunken neighbor.

The Uses of Compression in the Trailers for *Titus* and *Hamlet*

Trailers for films based on Shakespeare's plays are complicated by the cultural weight of the author's name. For some, that name will be enough to ensure attendance, but for most, it is something that must be compensated for: "Yeah, it's Shakespeare, but no one wears tights and there are explosions." One of the most important ways Hollywood trailers for Shakespeare films work is by focusing on the celebrities in the film. Instead of telling us who the characters are or about the conflict or the story, the trailer gives us the name and face of the film's stars. The celebrity faces carry the drama in miniature. The unconscious and instantaneous process of seeing Kenneth Branagh as Hamlet is a conceptual compression in the same way that seeing red as hot is. Celebrity faces and names anchor character creation and expose the unconscious process of compression.

Although casting celebrities in a Shakespeare play or film is derided as just a way to sell tickets, the practice operates as a powerful storytelling tool. As I have argued elsewhere, Michael Almereyda's casting of Sam Shepard as the Ghost of Ethan Hawke's father in his *Hamlet* (2000) tells a particular story of an old-world cowboy/astronaut being disappointed in his postmodern, slacker son:

> As the ghost of Hamlet's father, Shepard is the death of theater, replaced by a video artist who rents old movies to understand how to feel. He is crying for revenge to a son who we know will only disappoint him. He is the old west and high art looking to [a] disaffected New York arty intellectual for salvation. He is the past left homeless by the apathetic, postmodern present. Sam Shepard is only on screen for a few minutes, yet based on the mental spaces he evokes, he tells the story without speaking a word.[5]

The complicated relationship between father and son is conveyed through the shorthand of casting Hawke and Shepard; what spectators cannot follow in the poetry is staged in the ghosts of previous roles played by the actors.

The other brilliant casting choice in Almereyda's film is for the other father: Bill Murray as Polonius.[6] Whereas Shepard brings past roles as a tough, intelligent cowboy—as well as a real life persona as a playwright—Murray's roles prior to this film were almost exclusively comedic. He often played a depressed or damaged person in films strongly framed as comedies (*Ghostbusters* [1984], *What about Bob?* [1991], *Groundhog Day* [1993]). In Almereyda's *Hamlet*, Polonius becomes hilariously tragic. Murray's lack of serious roles prior to *Hamlet* meant that Almereyda could count on spectators bringing to the film an expectation that Polonius, as played by Murray, would be funny. That expectation meant that Murray didn't need to do anything funny; he simply provided a way of thinking about Polonius as funny, and indeed, Polonius can be very funny. Generally, because he is found in the midst of a tragedy, he is not an easy character to know you can laugh at. Although Bill Murray plays it deadly serious, his past means that we perceive the humor in his tying his daughter's shoes or going on at length about Hamlet's alleged madness. Casting a comic actor as Polonius might also invite the spectator to anticipate a happy ending—that is the trajectory of a comedy—an expectation dashed when Polonius is shot in the eye through Gertrude's closet door.[7]

Celebrity casting often works to evoke intertextuality, as many critics have noted. Lisa Starks analyzes Glenn Close's casting as Gertrude to Mel Gibson's Hamlet in terms of her most powerful previous role: "Glenn Close's physical presence in *Hamlet* derives significance from these contexts through the 'cinematic unconscious'—the intertextual meanings generated by Close's other roles, in such films as Adrian Lyne's *Fatal Attraction*. . . . Close's *Fatal Attraction* image as a 'hysterical, violent female' contributes significantly to the cultural and ideological meanings of the maternal in Zeffirelli's *Hamlet*."[8] Close, who was 43 at the time the movie was filmed, was only nine years older than Mel Gibson, who played her son Hamlet, which encouraged the spectators to perceive a potential sexual relationship between mother and son. Whether the Freudian reading of Zeffirelli's *Hamlet* comes from the age of the actors or intertextual meanings brought it by Close, it's the casting of the film that drives the interpretation.

Picking up on Keir Elam's call for a "post-semiotics of Shakespearean drama," Barbara Hodgdon asks, "How does 'character' get recited in relation to the body of a specific actor, inviting spectators to engage in a negotiation between actor and character? And how does that double body function as a locus for a spectator's imaginative desire to reperform the role?"[9] She finds in Ian McKellen's Richard in *Richard III* (1995) and Al Pacino's Richard in *Looking for Richard* (1996) moments when the actor's body, personal life, and personae are deeply implicated in the staging of these roles. Hodgdon argues that these filmic roles are a kind of "reply to their own previous performances."[10] McKellen's Richard, for example, recalls for the knowing spectator his revival at the National Theatre of his role of Max in *Bent* by Martin Sherman, a play famous for being one of the earliest to explicitly deal with gay themes. The revival occurred in reaction to anti-homosexual legislation and McKellen's public response:

> When *Richard III* opened in late July 1990, it also took shape within more insistently local theatrical and political conditions. In the late 1980s, Britain's Tory government had stigmatized homosexuality through passing Clause 28 of the Local Government code, legislation which precipitated McKellen, who had come out in 1988 on a BBC radio programme, into a more openly political stance. . . . In a Britain in which many freedoms had been eroded and in which the level of sexual intolerance was on the rise, the events *Bent* dramatizes had immediate resonances, and McKellen's performance as the character who initially disavows and then accepts his gay identity created an audience that, however temporarily, became engaged in queer activism.[11]

Thus, McKellen's body "doubles" the body of Richard, bringing the publically "out" McKellen onstage with the deformed Richard. Richard Loncraine's directorial choices highlight this doubling, in particular his staging a part of the famous opening soliloquy in a men's bathroom with McKellen/Richard using a urinal, audibly urinating while saying "but I that am not shaped for sportive tricks nor made to court an amorous looking glass, I that am rudely stamped." Hodgdon notes, "Never, I think, has a mainstream Richard taken quite as much bodily risk of exposing his private parts, however quickly they are covered up. . . . Is this body McKellen's or Richard's? Is he or isn't he? And what about the spectator? What is he (and especially she) doing there in the gents? Who, exactly, *is* the spectator being hailed in this film?"[12] Hodgdon's essay includes reviewer reactions, directorial choices, and comments by McKellen on the casting of the film as evidence that McKellen's "gay" body performs (in a Butlerian sense) in this film. Hodgdon cites Judith Butler's argument that such a performance can be subversive: "If men speak their homosexuality, that speaking threatens to bring into explicitness and, hence, destroy the homosociality by which the class of men coheres."[13] This is a powerful claim for performance and leaves me wondering how it is that a celebrity's body can show through and "perform" in one way or another.[14]

If celebrities operate as a way to communicate complicated story information in a Shakespeare play to a modern audience, then the trailer for a new Shakespeare film should maximize the visibility of the celebrities in the cast to increase the prospective audience's familiarity with and excitement about the production. Although *Titus* (1999) and *Hamlet* (1996) derive from very different plays and had very different directors (Julie Taymor in the first instance and Kenneth Branagh in the second), the trailers for both films tell a story through celebrity casting. Although *Hamlet* is perhaps burdened with too much popular exposure and *Titus Andronicus* is burdened with almost none, both trailers use the background information audience members have about the celebrities in the respective films to ensure that they know what they will get when they see the film. In three minutes, we know what we can expect from a three-hour film.

In hushed tones, the narrator of the trailer for Taymor's *Titus* (1999) starts out "For those who think revenge is sweet . . ." and then pauses as Anthony Hopkins plays with a knife as he taunts Chiron and Demetrius, who hang upside down like cattle for slaughter, with his plans to "grind their bones to dust."[15] The narrator then says "taste this" over a close-up of Hopkins snapping hungrily at the air. The trailer evokes the celebrity of Hopkins and his famous role as Hannibal Lecter with a close-up, using the familiar face to ease the burden of the unfamiliar text. Many viewers of this trailer would not have needed more than the image of knife-wielding Hopkins to be reminded of his Academy Award–winning performance in *The Silence of the Lambs* (1991), but the suggestion of his eating flesh will cement the recall. Hopkins himself referred to his performance of Titus as a mixture of Hannibal Lecter and King Lear. This frames *Titus* as a kind of sequel or spin-off. The audience connects the story from Hopkins's most well-known film with the less well-known play. The trailer prompts the information spectators have about the actor's previous roles—Hopkins as Hannibal—and historical information that may be available to them about Rome and war. We may know that Hopkins has been knighted or that he had recently played Richard Nixon, but this information recedes before other facts that dominate the trailer: his line of vicious text, his baring of his teeth, the "taste this" text of the narrator. Spectators of the trailer project information from what we know about Hopkins's most famous other part so that we create a new character around the spine of one who is already available to us. When the narrator gets to the "taste this" climax, the viewer can project the story of Hannibal as revenge-seeker onto the Roman backdrop and have a sense of what it is about: Hannibal Lecter started as a Roman soldier and was driven crazy by grief. This is a Shakespearean prequel.

What the trailer fails to show is equally important as what

it shows. It does not mention that Anthony Hopkins has been knighted or that he was nominated for an Academy Award for his portrayal of a reserved butler in *Remains of the Day* (1993). It does not linger on Hopkins's physical appearance or give us many lines from the play to explain who Titus is. There is very little Shakespearean dialogue and no mention of Shakespeare's name. The trailer does not focus on the other actors and does not name them. It focuses the viewer's attention on one element of the story and one element of the casting: the cooking and eating of people by Anthony Hopkins. After watching the film, however, one might be concerned with other moments of intertextuality, such as Taymor's casting of Alan Cumming as Saturninus because of his previous role in *Cabaret*. Samuel Crowl critiqued this as an unrealized attempt:

> Cumming came to Titus fresh from his award-winning performance in the revival of *Cabaret,* and one sees what must have struck Taymor about parallels between the demimonde world of 1930s Berlin and ancient Rome, but trying to link Saturninus with the Nazis and Fascists remains an idea poorly realized. . . . Cumming's Saturninus is an insipid brat who strikes poses.[16]

A Hollywood trailer is not likely to evoke a Broadway show for its audience, but there were certainly ways it could have done that. A director can offer an audience a simplified access point to his or her production by reducing the information a trailer presents and relying heavily on the information spectators bring.

The trailer for *Hamlet*, on the other hand, promotes a star-studded cast, telling a story through the celebrities in the film. While it may be true that, as the *New York Times* review of Branagh's film points out, *Hamlet* contains some of the most famous lines in the English language, it does not follow that the average filmgoer understands how those lines convey the plot or the relationships among the characters. Branagh relies heavily on the personae of the celebrity—instead of, or at least in addition to, their acting ability—to tell the story of the Danish prince in a rotten European capital. It starts with drumbeats, swords, soldiers on horses, and the screaming face of Kate Winslet as Ophelia. The first celebrity named is not William Shakespeare— although the narrator does say that the film is adapted from the "most celebrated drama of the English language"—but Kenneth Branagh, shown in his skull-holding pose with blond hair that evokes film's most famous Hamlet, Laurence Olivier. The narrator then mentions the "distinguished international cast" while showing the face of Robin Williams. For audience members who had seen him in *Birdcage* (1996) earlier that year or *Mrs. Doubtfire* (1993) a few years before, the question of how Robin Williams belonged in *Hamlet* seems a fair one. The narrator names the many stars as the screen displays each celebrity in costume but largely devoid of context: Robin Williams, Derek Jacobi, Billy Crystal, Charlton Heston, Jack Lemmon, Richard Attenborough, and John Gielgud. No matter how well you think you know *Hamlet*, you are forgiven for thinking you must have forgotten a few parts if all these celebrities fit into the same play. Even though two of the actors named above are famous for playing Hamlet, in this film, they are mostly playing small parts—or parts not even in the original play. Jack Lemmon plays Marcellus, a guard, in the first scene; Richard Attenborough plays an English ambassador; and John Gielgud plays Priam in a strange flashback scene that Branagh cuts to while the Player (Charlton Heston) gives his speech to the court. Janet Maslin of the *New York Times* calls the cast "so big-name and polyglot that it could be assembled almost as reasonably for a celebrity roast," but the analogy of an all-star game seems more appropriate to me: while these actors may be working together in the film, they haven't fully removed their regular "star" costumes.[17]

The narrator ends the cast list with "and Kenneth Branagh as Hamlet." At that point, the narration stops and the screen action begins; we see confetti falling in the castle as Claudius is crowned, a partially naked Branagh and Winslet in a made-up flashback scene, the sword fight, the murders, and the soldiers arriving with Fortinbras, and we hear the same music that un-

derscored Branagh's "band of brother's speech" in his successful film *Henry V* (1989). While the trailer hails Shakespeareans,
Branagh fans, and lovers of lush period films, the list of celebrities it presents suggests that we do not need to understand what
the actors are saying to know how we are to understand their
parts. Moreover, the trailer casts Branagh as the intellectual and
artistic force capable of bringing all these Hollywood and London celebrities together in England's most famous play.

Branagh's film extends the three minutes of the trailer into
a four-hour production that demonstrates the power and efficiency of casting celebrities in Shakespeare. Through his casting,
Branagh announces his intention to connect theatrical London
with filmic Hollywood. Charlton Heston plays the Player King
whom Hamlet warns not to "Out Herod Herod." Prompted by the
casting, the audience immediately understands that this Player
King could use Hamlet's directorial advice. Indeed, when Heston
hosted *Saturday Night Live* in 1987 and 1993, he spoofed his broad
acting style both times. With Heston's Moses from *The Ten Com-
mandments* in our minds, we know what "out Herod Herod" means
even if we have no formal knowledge of Roman history or Elizabethan theatrical practices. During the Player King's speech—
the one that inspires Hamlet to wonder how an actor can cry for
Hecuba when he can't cry for his father—Branagh shows foot-
age of Priam and Hecuba in action; the sequence functions like a
flashback that helps us understand what Heston is talking about.
Priam and Hecuba are played by Judi Dench and John Gielgud
and the comparison highlights Heston's acting. Dench and Gielgud's appearance is very brief and is not central to the plot, but
the casting of these two actors will richly reward some viewers.
Gielgud, cast as Priam, might be perceived as Branagh poking fun
at American actors who attempt to perform roles originated by
British actors, since Heston the Player King is so clearly unable
to capture Gielgud's performance of a king. Some viewers may
see in Gielgud the ghost of his Hamlet and wonder what it means
that Heston is representing the Gielgud "Hamlet" as a player in
an attempt to move or motivate Branagh's Hamlet.

By staging and casting these characters—characters that are not actually roles for actors in Shakespeare's play—Branagh is telling the story of the War of the Theatres in a different way to a different audience. Although Shakespeare's players provide Hamlet with the mechanism for catching the conscience of the King, they do not belong in the rotten world of Denmark; instead, they provide Shakespeare with an opportunity to refer to current affairs in his own theatrical universe. Hamlet calls upon the players to recite a speech that he had heard perhaps only once because it was "caviar to the general" and "pleas'd not the millions." Those comments would probably not have made sense to every member of the audience (and indeed, the part of the players was drastically reduced in the First Quarto), but a small portion of the audience would have been rewarded by getting Shakespeare's references to boy players sending professional companies into the countryside—and thus decreasing the work for the more "elite" actors and playwrights. They would know who Shakespeare referred to when they hear of a young actor being "cracked i' the ring," and thus unable to continue playing the female parts. Such metatheatrical moments furthered not only the spectator's understanding of *Hamlet* but also that person's experience in the Globe at that moment as one who was privy to inside information that enriched character players by displaying the players playing them. Branagh couldn't hope to make that clear to any of the audience for his film (except perhaps for the odd Shakespeare scholar), but he used casting to call our attention to the relationship between film and stage, London and Hollywood, by recasting Shakespeare's theatrical challenges with his own.[18]

Cameo Casting

The cameo role in film has offered directors and actors many opportunities to generate emergent structure. When the star is so much bigger than his part, the spectator's attention can be drawn to the making of the film, the power of the director, and the irony of the collision. The spectator who spots Peter Jackson in *The Lord of the Rings* film or Alfred Hitchcock in any of his films feels a part of the process; the film winks at him and unveils a metacommentary. Casting a big star in a small role may also allow the director to trust that the spectators will understand the character by referencing the celebrity; it is an effective directorial shorthand. Branagh casts Billy Crystal as the Gravedigger, and the audience immediately fills in what it doesn't know about the character with what it does know about the actor. We may not understand how the man digging Ophelia's grave is funny (Shakespeare's legal jokes do not help the humorless situation), but we trust that it is funny when we see Billy Crystal.[19] Similarly, when Crystal and Robin Williams play their personas in a Shakespeare film, they expand their "brand" and reify their "character."

Celebrities can also use cameos to complicate their personas. In Ben Stiller's *Tropic Thunder* (2008), Tom Cruise plays the character of Les Grossman, a fat, hairy, balding, abusive Hollywood producer. Cruise's filmography includes very few (if any) ugly or dislikable characters. When he wades into unlikeable territory (*Rain Man*, *Jerry Maguire*), the movie redeems him in the end. Some may not recognize Cruise in *Tropic Thunder* in his bald cap, fat suit, and large hairy fake hands, but the film adds gratuitous scenes of his dancing to prompt the spectator to wonder what the joke is. In addition to being funny because it is surprising to see Cruise so against character, it is also funny because once we know it is Cruise, we are laughing at the character along with the actor playing the character.[20] The character and the actor are pulled apart by the casting so that we can safely laugh at this idea of a man. Cruise removes the makeup and costume and is still Cruise, but now his persona includes this "risky" performance as an unlikeable man.[21]

The first definition of "cameo" in the *Oxford English Dictionary* is "a precious stone having two layers of different colours, in the upper of which a figure is carved in relief, while the lower serves as a ground," and while the editors of the dictionary say that it comes from the Italian, the original derivation is not known. A cameo sculpture distinguishes figure from ground through color and lines, creating an image out of differentiation. A cameo communicates by reducing the information that is given. The second definition of cameo relates the idea to language or narrative: "a short literary sketch or portrait; a small character part that stands out from the other minor parts." The first use of the term to refer to an actor in a film is in Edmund Crispin's *Frequent Hearses: A Detective Story* from 1950: "A cameo part . . . the film equivalent of a bit part on the stage." In film today, a cameo role is one in which the celebrity is bigger than the part, creating a kind of piercing of the narrative world by the outsized status of the star. Branagh casts stars in cameos in *Hamlet* to stage their personas, not the characters of the parts.

Names

Although trailers are a relatively new phenomenon, the need for a tool that can seduce and communicate through information reduction is not. Names are themselves compressions, ways of encapsulating a person with a tag. This tagging works efficiently to generate knowledge of a person's past and future. A name can be an interesting synecdoche; it can refer to the whole while mentioning only a part (as in "Junior" or "mom"). Names work cognitively to frame an interaction with a person or a thing. In John Macnamara's study of how we name things, he argues that naming "presupposes the power of distinguishing among objects" and that a name is a way of signifying importance. Based on experiments with children under the age of two, Macnamara concludes that "by the time he comes to learn vocabulary the child has learned not only to divide the world into classes, but to treat the individuality of the members of certain classes as important. The individuality of the members of most classes is usually not important."[22] A name labels and hails an individual in a class and often carries additional, compressed information.

Character names in Shakespeare carry a tremendous amount of information: from nobility status to character traits to casting. To be "of name" in Shakespeare is to have importance. Henry V motivates his men into battle by telling them that they may, if they outlive the day, be associated with the men of name with whom they fought. At the end of the battle, Henry reads the names of the nobles on the English side who have died and seems to shrug off the regular folks who fought with him on that day: "Where is the number of our English dead? / Edward the Duke of York, the Earl of Suffolk, Sir Richard Ketly, Davy Gam, esquire: / None else of name; and of all other men / But five and twenty" (4.8.95–98). Rafael Lyne points out how in *A Midsummer Night's Dream*, Bottom, a character named for a tool of his trade (and for his personality) "adapts with admirable ingenuity" when he awakes among the fairies, having been turned into a literal ass:

> He starts by asking for the fairies' names with an exaggerated tone of respect. The names give him something to work with. . . . Bottom does not really achieve a significant apprehension of his surroundings, but his puns and associations serve a basic heuristic purpose. They enable him to interact and to become part of a social situation, which is a meaningful achievement.[23]

However, as Lyne points out, Bottom simply presumes that the naming system that labels him in reference to his social position (as a weaver) also applies to the fairy world. Thus, he thinks that he knows something about the fairies when he knows their names. As Lyne's rich reading has it: "His cognitive rhetoric, accordingly, is based on simple analogies and word-play, rather than on tropes that entail a conceptual shift that could actually offer insight."[24] To know a name is to be given a clue about the social system that names, and Bottom failed to understand this.

Murray J. Levith, who examines the system of naming at work in Shakespeare's plays, points out how when "dealing with minor and especially comic characters and secondary play actions, Shakespeare will single out a vivid attribute and so label a character, either by occupation, physical trait or feature, or some notable aspect of personality." So "Malvolio is ill-willed and Benvolio is good-willed in keeping with their names" and Nym, the friendly pickpocket of *Henry V* and *The Merry Wives of Windsor*, has a name that means to steal.[25] As Levith notes, "Such allusion serves oftentimes to delineate character rapidly or may have a comic function."[26] Having a name that announces character gives us less to remember: name and trait are combined and thus the name primes the associated trait and the performance of the trait then reminds us of the name. Further, it aids in anticipation: hearing that Fortinbras is at the gates seems ominous, whereas being arrested by someone named Elbow does not seem very threatening. Just as what seeing Billy Crystal's face does for contemporary audiences, hearing a name in a Shakespeare play can tell us what to expect from that character. Shakespeare uses names to help this categorization, giving his characters names that communicate personality (Malvolio, Benvolio, Dogberry), refer to geographic regions of England (Westmoreland, Gloucester, Exeter), or evoke tales memorized at school (Ganymede, Titus, Lavinia).

In *Titus Andronicus*, Lavinia's fate is foretold in her name. Just as modern-day viewers knew that Titus was going to be involved in some kind of cannibalistic darkness from the first moment they saw Anthony Hopkins's face, an early modern audience would bring to the play certain expectations about Lavinia's character from her name. Levith tells the story of the name Lavinia from Virgil's *Aeneid*: "Despite a previous betrothal, she is promised to Aeneas by her father, and thus becomes the innocent cause of much anguish."[27] Jonathan Bate explains the historical context of her name in *Titus Andronicus* as "Virgil's Lavinia, the mother of early Rome, [who] becomes the mutilated daughter of late Rome."[28] Lavinia is referred to by her name twenty times in the short time that she is onstage before being raped. The tale foretold by her name is enacted even before act one is complete: even though she is betrothed to Bassianus, her father gives her to Saturninus. At the start of act two, Aaron connects her to Lucrece ("Lucrece was not more chaste / Than this Lavinia, Bassianus' love") and her fate becomes patterned by that of a wife of later Rome. Aaron then mentions the third precedent for Lavinia's fate, Philomel, a woman in Greek mythology who was raped by her sister's husband. Before killing his daughter, Titus asks Saturninus to give his opinion on another legal precedent: "Was it well done of rash Virginius / To slay his daughter with his own hand, / Because she was enforced, stained and deflowered?" (5.3.36–8). From the moment she is introduced in the play—"Gracious Lavinia, Rome's rich ornament" (1.1.55)—the character of Lavinia points to a larger story. Just like the "tedious sampler" on which Philomel "sew'd her mind," these stories are compressed down to the pattern meant to predict or inspire current and future action, reaction, and revenge.

Although in fiction we rarely have to keep track of different people with the same names, in real life we often know more than one Amy or more than one John. The way to make naming simple would be for all of us to have different words to identify ourselves. If there were no other Amys in the world, we would never have to explain which one we meant. However, if everyone had to have a unique identifier, our language would be multiplied to such an extent as to be completely unmanageable. There are major historical differences between the early modern period and our times in terms of the number of names in circulation. As Michael Ramscar and his collaborators have shown, industrialization increased the number of different names in circulation. In 1600, "50% of boys born in England were named William, John or Thomas," but in the twentieth century, there was "a big decline in the number of babies being given the most frequent names, and an increase in the diversity of given names."[29] My son's second grade class had an Equin, an Atticus, and a Titus, but no William, John, or Thomas. Surnames once helped link us to our family (Donaldson), our geographic region (of Orange), our appearance (Whitehead), or our job (Farmer), and thus we could be located categorically, if not individually. Names then were like a suitcase handle, facilitating the movement and use of a lot of information (they still are). The system a culture uses to handle names has implications for its functioning, because a greater diversity in individual identifiers makes it more difficult to remember the right name.

Our name, then, acts like a casting device, giving others a shorthand or sketch of who we may (or may not) be. Some names are tainted with the memory of a predecessor. In some cases, the memory might be personal—the horrible kid who bullied you in third grade shares the name with your friend's new boyfriend—and in other cases, it is universal—it may be legal to name your kid Adolph Hitler Campbell, but you will have difficulty getting a birthday cake made for him.[30] When Princess Kate and Prince William announced that she was pregnant with the second royal baby, British bookmakers were already tallying the odds for the likely name. Among those given odds were Caledonia and Macbeth (both 500 to 1), Nigel (100 to 1), Charlotte (12 to 1), and James (6 to 1).[31] Though the royal couple has a bit more freedom to name the "spare," the name of the heir was circumscribed by history and the child's future. They could not have named their firstborn son Nigel or Macbeth. Nigel is not the name of a king. Shakespeare would never have named Kate and William's baby Nigel.

There are only so many things we can keep track of in our world, and the more we compress, the more we can think about. Evelyn Tribble describes the necessity of cognitive thrift in the theater of Shakespeare and argues that breaking the play into the "parts" enables compression and efficiency: "Parts isolate the most important (*salient*) elements of the play for each actor and minimize mnemonic burdens by stripping all unnecessary information, facilitating information 'underload.'"[32] In making predictions about the behavior of others, we compress our previous experience with them into traits that we then use to read their current behavior. This allows us to be efficient, but it is not always accurate or fair. Character attributes provide us with a way of quickly and efficiently perceiving continuity in a person so we can manage our attention to them and our memory of them.

Psychological studies have found interesting ways that we cast people as certain types. Psychologist Richard Gerrig and colleagues have argued that people tend to create an inner quality to explain an outer trait. These "dispositional attributions" are what lead us to see Jane's cheating on the test as a result of her being a liar and John's helping to clean up the mess because he's kind, even when there's very little evidence that the action and the trait are related. "What this suggests, as a start, is that people bring to their experiences of narratives well-practiced processes that derive dispositional explanations for characters' behavior."[33] Gerrig and colleagues claim that experience with literary narratives reinforces this tendency: "literary characters (as captured by trait descriptions) provide a type of consistency that is not, in fact, present in everyday experiences."[34] As we read Jane Austen, Shakespeare, or Ian Fleming, we keep track of individuals by generating expectations of their actions based on our initial experience with them and then viewing the action that ensues as being inevitable, given the characters involved. In a different study, Gerrig and David W. Allbritton argue that "differential attention and memory go a long way toward explaining why different people develop mutually exclusive impressions of the same individuals. We color objectively neutral information to fit our initial hypothesis."[35] In other words, we quickly—though not necessarily accurately—generate assumptions about the traits of others and then perceive future information in light of this initial trait.

Suzanne Keen calls for reader-response studies that are "informed by the evidence of the high degree of variability in reactions to fictional characters."[36] For Keen, these differences change how we construct characters: "The cognitivists suggest that we bring along and contribute knowledge structures to our reading of character; indeed, we do far more than that, when as embodied readers we rehearse our own temperaments in our responses to fictional character."[37] Although there is disagreement about the degree to which this rehearsal happens,[38] Keen's point is that reading is not a disembodied process and that our experience with and through our own bodies not just informs our reading of character but in fact *is* our experience of character. Character categorization is embodied, rather than symbolic, and thus keeping Osric discerned from Hamlet discerned from Laertes leverages information that is dispersed across the body. How the character moves, for example, may register in the spectator's motor system and generate assumptions or predictions about the character even if the spectator is not consciously aware of the physical response or its consequences. This dispersed information can be compressed into a sketch or a name or a gesture so that we can efficiently keep track of many characters in our lives and on our stages.

Naming and categorizing provides a linguistic scaffolding that shapes and builds our minds. The first block in the linguistic structure is labeling: "mama," "dada," "doggy." Teaching a baby to name is giving them power. In *Supersizing the Mind: Embodiment, Action, and Cognitive Extension*, Andy Clark argues that this naming, or "tagging," allows us to offload cognitive tasks. He points to a study about a chimp that was trained to understand numerals. Despite this understanding, when the chimp was shown two plates of treats (one with more than the other) and asked to point to the one her friend should get, she would point to the bigger one, even though it gave her fewer treats. However, when they labeled the plates with the number of treats on them, she was able to choose the smaller number to give to her friend, leaving herself the plate with the larger number of treats. Tagging, the researchers hypothesize, enabled her to override the complicated information about lots of treats into information she could assess. This "reduce[d] the descriptive complexity of the scene" and made thinking about the choice possible.[39] Clark extends this to sentences and ideas, arguing that once we make an idea into a written thought, we can see and manipulate it. We can see this with personification: a set of culturally valued traits can be given a name, "virtue," and then given a female shape, "Virtue," so that we can think about her, it, or them.[40] We could extend this to stories, allegories, and performances: we stage an idea to interact with it. Because we are embodied and embedded cognitive agents, something must be an "it" before we can think about it, so we give names to "objects" and create something out of "airy nothing."

The Face(s) that Launched a Thousand Ships

In the beginning of western theatrical time, a face launched a ship that burned down a town. Well, before that there was a curse on the House of Atreus, but Menelaus and Agamemnon (brothers in the house of Atreus) went to war because the Trojan Paris took Helen from Menelaus. In Christopher Marlowe's famous mighty line at the end of *Doctor Faustus*, Helen's face can be read as a synecdoche of her whole person (or even more broadly, the person's relationship with Paris) or it could be that it was her face by *itself* that won Paris's love and inspired him to take her from Menelaus back to Troy, which prompted Menelaus to secure his own forces as well as Agamemnon's and motivated Artemis to call upon Agamemnon to murder his daughter Iphigenia in order to bring the winds that allowed him to finally launch the ships that set sail for Illium with the many soldiers who then burned those topless towers. Marlowe did not need to investigate the chain of events that led to the destruction of Troy; he simply needed to refer to her face. The line is a blend in which cause and effect are connected (her face as cause is connected to the launching and the burning) while omitting (through compression) the actual agents (most notably the men who did the sailing and the fighting and the burning). What this both generates and reflects is the power of the face to anchor character and cognition. Just like we think of the character of Hannibal Lecter when we see Hopkins's teeth-baring face, Helen's face anchors us to the whole character and the whole story. Of course, Helen was nowhere near the ships that set sail to retrieve her from Paris and she played no part in the burning of Troy. For Faust, though, it started with her face.

The face is more than one of the parts of the body; the face is what we call the person. We page through a photo album or a magazine and point to the faces ("there's my grandmother," "there's Leonardo DiCaprio") without confusing the living, breathing person with her or his image. The face is a compression of the person to a part. We also do not need more than the face to identify our grandmother or Leonardo DiCaprio. If we found a photograph of a leg or an arm we would not say "who is that?"; we might say "whose arm is that?" A photograph of a face *is* the character, despite all the ways in which it is not the person. A photograph does not breathe or move or make rational decisions. A photograph of the face, however, prompts the construction of the character in our minds, not the biological realities of the person. From shortly after birth, babies track the faces of their caregivers and demonstrate preferential looking at a new face. Our language reflects the degree to which social interaction privileges the face—"we met face to face," "he wouldn't say it to my face"—and even helps us organize the world around us—"the face of the mountain was daunting." When we refer to the "face" of a company, we are talking in compressed form about the person who has the authority to represent the entire company—Rupert Murdoch, Steve Jobs. The face presents the character of the company. The face, like the name, gives us a character anchor.[41] The process by which we compress and categorize a whole into a more manageable part is similar to the process we use to unite the factors of casting into a unit that facilitates and encourages interaction. The casting director might match actor to character, but the spectator watching the film builds the character through that casting in much the same way that the brain works with new and old faces. The research on how we process faces and what happens when we fail to process them gives us a way to understand casting not just as a creative matching between actor type and character type but also as a cognitive process of categorization.

Facial recognition in humans is so specialized that most of us can recognize familiar faces almost instantly even when they are presented without hair, clothes, or other identifiers. But some of us can't, and that's also how we know how specialized the ability is. People with prosopagnosia are "face blind"; they cannot recognize people they know very well from seeing their faces. The artist Chuck Close, who produces large, up-close paintings of faces, cannot recognize the faces of the people he sees. He has to flatten them to two dimensions in order to study them. The scientist Oliver Sacks was also face blind; he wrote lovely portraits of his patients but could not recognize them on the street. Sacks once even mistook another man for a reflection of himself. One woman who has a head injury that damaged her facial recognition center and can no longer recognize people, including her family and even herself, said, "It's kind of like I've lost everybody, like everybody is gone. All I'm really left with is facts without faces."[42] Perhaps seeing the "facts without the faces" contributed to Close's art and Sack's science; perhaps their deficit enabled them to complicate the person, to unblend people from their faces. The efficient and useful connection between the facts of a face and the person, such that "mom" or "Chuck" *is* the face, is missing or is damaged in people with prosopagnosia.

Being able to recognize the difference between one person and another is useful in life and pivotal in theater and film. As difficult as narratives can be to follow, imagine what it would be like if you simply could not perceive any difference in the faces of Hamlet, Horatio, and Laertes. Or Bond, M, and Dr. No. Not everyone with prosopagnosia is completely face blind; Richard Russell and his colleagues study a range of deficits. They refer to "developmental prosopagnosics," who "report not having much interest in film or television, because their inability to recognize the different characters makes it difficult to follow the story."[43] Processing narrative performance relies on our ability to quickly recognize and connect face to character.

The experience of watching narrative performance (film, theater, television) is also different for those who are incredibly good at face recognition, or "super-recognizers." These people can recognize a near-total stranger after years of not seeing them. "All report being able to recognize actors playing minor characters or 'extras' in movies, television, and advertisements from other roles they have played."[44] For super-recognizers, the connection between face and identity is so strong that it holds up maybe too well, making it harder for them to perceive actors as disappearing into a new character. Although this specific research has not been done, the relationship between facial recognition and character tracking suggests that a certain amount of strategic forgetting facilitates the tracking of fictional characters on screen.

Most people find it harder to recognize an object if it is displayed upside down. This "inversion effect" is significantly greater when people try to recognize faces than when they try to recognize other inverted objects.[45] For prosopagnosics, the "face inversion effect" is greatly diminished; they are just as bad at recognizing the face right side up as upside down. For super-recognizers, though, the "face inversion effect" is greater: seeing a face upside down significantly reduces their ability to recognize it.[46] The perception of faces is a specialized phenomenon, and making sense of faces, discerning between different faces, is central to our ability to track and categorize the people in our lives.

Some faces also elicit an emotional response. When scientists show subjects a series of photographs of random people and the subject's mother, the image of mom generates a galvanic skin response. In other words, seeing mom's face makes you sweat. In fairness, subjects generated an emotional response (as measured in galvanic skin responses) to many familiar faces.[47] In some rare cases, however, individuals have lost the connection between the limbic system and the visual cortex. They can still recognize faces but fail to feel a reaction to them. They report that their mother (or father or spouse) may look like their mother (or father or spouse) but is in fact an imposter. This is called Capgras delusion (named for the French psychiatrist who identified it in the 1920s). These individuals will recognize the voice of their loved one over the phone, but visual stimuli do not evoke the feeling of the person for them. According to V. S. Ramachandran and Sandra Blakeslee, the lack of an emotional response to the loved one is so troubling that the patient confabulates a reason for the change: "The absence of this glow is therefore surprising and [the patient's] only recourse then is to generate an absurd delusion—to rationalize it or to explain it away."[48] If the recognition of mom is not there when the person sees mom's face, then this must not be mom. Hadyn Ellis and Michael Lewis point out that "simply a lack of automatic response is not itself sufficient to produce the Capgras delusion"; there must also be a "second-stage abnormality, perhaps within an attribution stage following face processing." Or perhaps "fronto-ventromedial lesioned patients still experience the affective response to familiar faces but there is still some interruption between this stage of processing and the processes causing changes in [skin conductance responses]."[49] Whatever the cause, we have developed a complicated system for binding facial stimuli to memories of whole individuals and an automatic emotional response to some of those individuals. Damage to any part of this system radically disrupts our ability to make sense of the characters in our lives.

We also have particular responses to the faces of celebrities. These faces circulate so constantly that we recognize them quickly and easily, even though most of us have no personal experience with them. Neurological studies of facial recognition suggest that your response to some important faces—your mother, your father, Jennifer Aniston—triggers highly specific neuronal firing patterns in the fusiform gyrus, the part of the brain that links to neural networks associated with recognition. Itzhak Friend was operating on an epileptic patient when he discovered what he came to call the "Jennifer Aniston Neuron," the single neuron that flashed only when the patient was shown a picture of Jennifer Aniston, any picture of Jennifer Aniston. In a story for NPR, Robert Krulwich jokingly condensed the theory:

Maybe the neuron flashing "Jennifer!" isn't acting alone. Maybe it's the beacon atop a summit of associated neurons, each of which is flashing little bits of Jen. After all, when I say Jennifer Aniston, what comes to mind? Her blue eyes. Her chin (I'm slayed by her chin), her hair of course, her voice, her laugh, her fictive romance with Ross on "Friends," her dresses at the Oscars, her marriage to Brad Pitt, the divorce, her movies. And more fundamentally, those Jen-parts are themselves built from rawer bits: the blue of her eyes, her smooth skin, her flowing hair, her facial patterns (especially chins), which are in turn made of even smaller bits: units of light, dark, color, shading, form. Those lower-down neurons are no doubt doing other things in my brain (blue-ing up skies, lakes, and other people's blue eyes) when they're not building Ms. Aniston, but when Aniston calls, they come.[50]

His tone suggests a connection between Aniston's attractiveness and the neuronal excitation that is misleading, but the description of a neuron that yokes together the firings of other neurons to "make up" Jennifer Aniston for us is useful. It is her familiarity rather than her beauty that activates this special neuron. Further research has shown that the more familiar the face, the more neurons will fire when presented with that face.[51] Research has suggested that the neuron fires in response to a broader concept of "Jennifer Aniston" instead of responding only to her face: "Our brains may use a small number of concept cells to represent many instances of one thing as a unique concept—a sparse and invariant representation."[52] The efficient compression that allows the brain to connect various elements of a concept (or a person) to one neuron is similar to the casting that yokes a character to an actor. Our brains cast important people in our lives by connecting their face to their identity with a particular efficiency. Your best friend could get a haircut and change her clothes—or her age—and you would still respond with trust, the recognition that you were home.

The face has often been the focal point of performance. In the Greek drama of Aeschylus, Sophocles, and Euripides, there were few characters and even fewer actors. Characters were recognized based on their masks, not the actors playing them. Masks have been powerful tools in performance across time and cultures because of the way they compress and convey so much

about character. John Emigh, who explored demon and apot-
ropaic masks and mask-like images from around the world, identified a particular facial expression that seems almost universally
to represent the demonic. "Bulging eyes, full lips, flared nostrils,
bared fangs, and, frequently, distended tongues" can be found in
representations such as a "Tasmanian Devil" in a film, Balinese
performance masks, and Maori ritual expressions.[53] Emigh suggests that perhaps it is the particular blend of human and bestial
features that makes the masks so evocative. Emigh described a
connection between a particular embodied experience of looking at the mask of a demon—tracking the absurdly oversized
features—and the ritual performance of the devil: we see in the
face an extreme figure of desire, of heightened sensation, man-
ifesting a kind of feared inner demon. Is it possible that mask
performance practices the important daily experience of tracking and making sense of faces?

It is precisely the face of the demon that we see in the trailer
for *Titus*: the bulging eyes and bared fangs of Hopkins's face. In
the past, masks circulated widely in performance, transforming
different performers into the same universally recognized creature. Like the masks of the past, contemporary media consumers return to the same celebrity faces again and again, comforted
by the familiar and released from effort because we so quickly
recognize a complex and abstract idea (evil) in simplified phys-
iognomy. The research on face recognition suggests that our
perception of faces involves highly specific neural networks and
that these trigger more than just the face. The face anchors story,
character, past, and anticipated future.

Casting involves a process of compression, efficiency, power,
and complexity that is similar to the cognitive process involved
in face recognition. How a film is cast shapes the thinking that
is possible with and through that film in the same way that the
degree to which we recognize a person's face influences the behavior called for by an interaction with that face. Familiar faces generate a kind of cognitive affection. A familiar face may be
comforting even when it is a devil face because of the speed with

which we know how to respond to the face. Seeing mom or Anthony Hopkins or George Clooney or Jennifer Aniston or even the Tasmanian devil allows us to process the environment more quickly because that face elicits a limited number of behaviors. So we swoon over Clooney, shiver when we see the devil, or relax with a friend.

Richard Maxwell, a downtown New York City theater director, explains character building to beginner actors far more simply than all that I have discussed in terms of compression:

> The character you play is the audience member's sum of what you say and do on stage. You say something, you do something (you wear something), and the viewers respond with their imagination. On stage, you're a "cocaine dealer" in the viewer's mind because you say you are. You're a 'dancer' because you're wearing leg-warmers. You are a 'bank robber' because you're seen heading out the door of 'the bank" carrying a duffel bag full of money. . . . Granted, if you are a beanpole, and on stage you only say you a bodybuilder, I'm less likely to register that label than if you say you're a bodybuilder and pick up a dumbbell and start working out. I might laugh, I might scratch my head, but I'm left with little choice but to believe it, since you put the idea in my head, and since I am cognizant of a story being told.[54]

Humans build characters with the information we are given; we are character-building and narrative-constructing creatures. Sometimes the characters are simply "dancer" and others are more complicated, but compression allows us to make sense of both within the narrative frame. In her examination of the celebrity casting of Shylock in the eighteenth century, Emily Hodgson Anderson looks at elements of eighteenth-century theater that made it possible for audiences to think of characters as separate from the actors who portrayed them. Hodgson points out how Samuel Taylor Coleridge and Charles Lamb both suggested that Shakespeare's "plays are better read than seen . . . since casting choices represent exercises in interpretation that threaten to foreclose future imaginings. For these critics, Shakespearean characters as staged [were] inevitably disappointing, because no one could suitably embody such complicated roles."[55] In the eighteenth century, to embody was to foreclose, to reduce the complexity of a character.

Casting is a form of dimensionality reduction: we reduce the astonishing complexity of the world around us by casting particular faces in particular roles. How we interact with these characters once they are cast in our lives is dynamic. Once we cast Anthony Hopkins as Titus or Branagh as Hamlet, we compress all the stimuli that constitute Hopkins and selectively project the elements that fit Titus. It is dynamic, though, because Hopkins does not disappear; his previous role becomes highly visible as soon as his character wields a chef's knife and serves Tamora her sons for dinner. We rely on compression to facilitate narrative comprehension, converting a weather pattern into a disorderly drunk, but we also play in the network dynamically. Compression is visible whenever we call out a name and expect the person to answer to that name. It is visible when we point to a face and talk about a memory of a relationship. It is visible when we turn Robin Williams into Osric and when we see Osric as also partially Mrs. Doubtfire.

CHAPTER 2

BUILDING CHARACTERS
Seeing Bodies

In an interview on *Fresh Air*, Dave Davies asked Maggie Smith where she found the inspiration for the Dowager Countess, her character on *Downton Abbey*. She credited the words: "mainly the way it was written by Julian [Fellowes], which was terrific, you know, and the wonderful lines to say. And it was written so elegantly."[1] It is lovely and generous of her to credit the writer in a situation where the interviewer may have been presuming that there might be an alternate inspiration for the character than the words. The only credit she took was for acting her age: "But it was quite funny because as I got up in this scene to say something to Penelope [Wilton], and I had my stick, and I was sort of doing that awful teetering and crouching about. And I said to Penelope why—why am I acting old? . . . It's the one thing I don't need to act."[2] Maggie Smith knew that her age and the words of the script would build the character, whether or not she was inspired. In the last chapter, I argued that spectators build characters from associations compressed and connected—a character's age, the script, previous roles played by the actor, etc. In this chapter, I argue that some information is more visible than others. This is the information that the actor doesn't need to act and often cannot mask.

While watching a performance, a spectator connects many pieces of information to build a character: the words written by the playwright or screenwriter, any historical knowledge a spectator has about the character or other versions of the story or character type, physical information about the actor, background information spectators have about the actor, and information spectators get from the other characters surrounding the character. This chapter looks at why some actors seem to "disappear" into their roles and others do not. Although this disappearance is often highly praised as the accomplishment of the actor, I argue that character building by spectators means that some bodies seem more rightly cast as some characters than others. By shifting the critical lens from the actor to the spectators for whom he or she performs, I locate character building where celebrity, actor, talent, story, and society combine.

Celebrity

Many academic discourses have examined the topics of celebrities and fame. Everyone wants to understand this form of power. How does one person command our attention when others do not? Why do we give so much of our time and money to noticing what they wear and seeing them drop off dry cleaning just like us? Why are we willing to pay so much more to see a celebrity in a play than another actor of equal or greater talent? I will draw on some of the answers to these questions that celebrity studies offers in order to assess the role that celebrity plays in building character. Celebrity is the inevitable result of visible character building; when a presence is visible to spectators over and over, when he or she seems to defy our categorizing, that presence can gain celebrity.

Celebrity studies is based on the idea that there are characters that come before the celebrities that enact them. Leo Braudy defines stars as those "who, for better or worse, represent some heightened form of human character."[3] In *The Frenzy of Renown*, Braudy explores the history of fame, arguing that "the modern preoccupation with fame is rooted in the paradox that, as every

advance in knowledge and every expansion of the world popula-
tion seems to underline the insignificance of the individual, the
ways to achieve personal recognition have grown corresponding-
ly more numerous."[4] In other words, celebrities are the inevitable result of our growing need for more "heightened form[s] of
human character." This presupposes that there is a human character, of course, that celebrities "heighten." In *Heavenly Bodies*,
Richard Dyer says, "Stars articulate what it is to be a human being in contemporary society."[5] They are the boiled-down essence
of the dispersed, pale fantasies of the many. Marilyn Monroe
became this "emblematic figure" in the 1950s, according to Dyer,
in large part due to the increased attention paid to sex and sexuality at the time and her ability to be both highly sexual and
innocent or even vulnerable. Monroe's genius, then, is partially
hers and partially an accident of history: if she didn't come along
at that time, audiences would have invented her. Sharon Marcus
then sees celebrity

> as a form of authorship, but a kind of authorship that dissolves the
> distinctions between original and copy on which both the Romantic
> notion of authorship and the legal regime of copyright were based.
> A form of authorship *intensified* by copying rather than vitiated or
> compromised by it; the copies generated by typification confer dis-
> tinction. Arguments against the kind of proprietary authorship de-
> fined by copyright usually contrast it to creation by the commons.
> Celebrity is interesting because rather than simply displace author-
> ship from the individual level to a collective one, it intensifies indi-
> viduality.[6]

Monroe gains individuality as she multiplies. But she also requires duplication and citation: "To be sure, even as celebrity
confects a fantasy about peerless, inimitable presence, it turns
individuality into a tissue of citations, since not only are stars
widely copied, they often present themselves as copies: Lady
Gaga echoes Madonna echoing Marilyn echoing Jean Harlow;
Wilde echoed Byron echoing Brummel."[7] So celebrity here seems

to point to what cannot ever have been: a character forever slipping from our grasp but only possible here and now by this manifestation.

Celebrities hold attention because they reference an impossible original; the character we never knew we needed. Celebrity studies, then, might question the making of character. In her essay "Celebrity Shylock," Emily Anderson Hodgson interrogates the portrayal of Shylock in the eighteenth-century, arguing that audiences responded both to the character and the actor, reading the famous character through the body of Charles Macklin, the actor, and then Macklin in reference to the character he played. She insists, "In thinking about how a dramatic character acquires celebrity and what that celebrity consists of, we need to consider how the models for celebrity studies and character criticism become not merely analogous but superimposed."[8] Shylock might be an example of what Linda Charnes's calls a *Notorious Identity*, characters—such as Shakespeare's Cleopatra and Richard III— who "exceed the reputations that always already precede them."[9] Charnes argues that the Shakespearean subject is materialized through this excess, where notoriety and character intersect. For Charnes, Cleopatra exceeds any attempt to "boy her." In other words, it is a role that far exceeds any attempt to be played. In this way, Shakespeare's notorious characters contain the future of their attempts to be captured:

> Drama, as written script that is repeatedly performable, embodies a principle of multiplicity, since it takes figures from narrative genres and "translates" them into dramatic figures, who are multiplied again by the actors who perform them, and yet again by subsequent performances with different actors. Consequently, Shakespeare's notorious characters are both finished and unfinished, absolute in what they "mean" yet multiplicitous in how that meaning is produced.[10]

These notorious characters may fail to write their own identity, but the embodiment of them—by Elizabeth Taylor, Al Pacino,

Ian McKellen—allows the actor to demonstrate this failure, holding together this intricate network of associations the spectator brings to the narrative. In this web, at this intersection, the spectator builds a character that contains multitudes.

Celebrities that have "it," that added something that makes certain actors impossible to look away from—Clara Bow, Clark Gable, Marlon Brando—capture our attention by remaining dynamic, not just one thing. According to Joseph Roach, "It" is

> the power of apparently effortless embodiment of contradictory qualities simultaneously: strength and vulnerability, innocence and experience, and singularity and typicality among them. . . . It comes out in the play of suddenly reversible polarities. Like a gestalt switch, during which the vase transforms itself, in the blink of the beholder's eye, into two faces juxtaposed, only to switch back again, reversible polarities appear both to cause It and to assert themselves as its most startling and continuously compelling effect."[11]

Clara Bow may be the original "It" girl; this quality exists in the eyes of her beholders. This "play of suddenly reversible polarities" is historically contingent: what a twentieth-century audience perceived as It is probably different from what a nineteenth-century audience perceived as It. The spectators find in It a cognitive workout, a category expander—an ingénue with grit, experience, and innocence—and they cannot look away because they are not done making sense of it. This is the cognitive work of the spectator and speaks to a cognitive hunger, as well as historical and cultural factors. Roach's It and his idea of surrogation—the replacement of one social or cultural need with another—are nouns, and his anatomization of these cultural phenomena is brilliant; but the process by which they occur—or where or how they occur—is unclear. In order for a celebrity to have It, there must be an audience capable of perceiving and appreciating the precious paradox—the sexuality and vulnerability, the strength and wound—that holds together in this person. There is no such thing as a celebrity in the forest. Spectators are hungry for these bodies who visibly muddy the narrative by conveying contradictory ideas at the same time.

Celebrities don't have to have "It" to conduct our attention. Many of them, of course, have extraordinary talent and technique, but even so it is often the fact of their celebrity that draws attention and drives ticket sales. Talent in acting is often equated with a celebrity's ability to "disappear" into a role—and more on this later—but celebrities don't sell tickets because they disappear but because they appear in certain ways and not others. Tom Cruise, Sir Anthony Hopkins, and Billy Crystal all prompted expectations by rendering visible one horizon of expectations about a character and forestalling another; Billy Crystal is making a joke and Tom Cruise is not the villain. Mike Nichol's production of Harold Pinter's *Betrayal*, with Daniel Craig and Rachel Weisz, broke box office records on Broadway. Although Craig was best known for playing James Bond, Pinter's play about a marriage struggling with infidelity brought attention to the fact that Craig and Weisz are married. Ben Brantley's review begins: "So just how sexy is it? Oh, admit it. That's the biggest question on your mind. You didn't pay all that money for tickets to "Betrayal" because it was written by the Nobel Prize-winning playwright Harold Pinter, the great master of existential dread and the vagaries of memory." He trusts that Craig's Bond reputation has something to do with it, but also, "It doesn't hurt that Mr. Craig is playing opposite his real-life wife, the beautiful, Oscar-winning movie star Rachel Weisz. Or that the subject of the play, at least on its most literal level, is marital infidelity."[12] Audiences of this production of *Betrayal* were stimulated by the complexity of multiple marriages, multiple possible characters, and multiple layers at the same time—like Roach's gestalt switch. Even without "It," the mathematics of celebrity, actor, characters, and narrative excite spectators. Craig and Weisz in these roles do not need Pinter's Nobel prize winning writing to interest us in a sexy married couple—we bring that to the theatre.

The cognitive power and efficiency of celebrities—heightened humans, category prototypes—make them very visible in narratives. This can enrich or weaken the experience, depending on casting. James Gandolfini played Tony Soprano on HBO's popular and award-winning TV Show *The Sopranos* from 1999 to 2007. Although it was hardly his first role, he was not known for any part in particular before he portrayed Tony, the mafia don with psychological issues, but he became highly celebrated for it. *The Sopranos* was one of the most influential TV shows in history, and Gandolfini's obituaries often echoed *The Hollywood Reporter*'s sentiments: "It's a terrible loss for the acting world. Gandolfini was memorable in pretty much everything he did but will forever be seen as Tony Soprano. It was a role he completely inhabited, a hulking presence able to project menace and kindness in equal measures."[13] Two years after the series finale of *The Sopranos*, Spike Jonze cast Gandolfini as Carol in his film of Maurice Sendak's popular children's book, *Where the Wild Things Are*. He played the erratically violent Thing that takes in the runaway Max and makes him king of the Wild Things. These Things are big and have all the teeth and claws that Sendak gave them in the book, but they are also furry and soft, like large fierce stuffed animals. As Manohla Dargis of the *New York Times* points out, "they have partly been brought to waddling life by performers in outsize costumes. (The fluid tremors of emotion enlivening the fuzzy faces were primarily created through computer-generated animation.) The vexed, whining, caressing voices . . . do the expressive rest."[14] Although we never see his face, James Gandolfini's voice brings a part of Tony Soprano to the Monstrous Thing.

This character comes together for the spectator in the network of a dispersed set of information. Sendak's book, which came out in 1963, has sold 19 million copies worldwide. Thus, it is safe to assume that many people in the audience for Jonze's film have previous knowledge of the book. In the book, Max's time with the Wild Things lasts only a page or two. He is threatened by them, he tames them, they make him their king, and they have a wild rumpus. Then Max returns home. We do not get to know the individual creatures and they do not have names. Because children's books are often read over and over, they allow kids to process the present in light of the past: once the book has been read the first time, we know that Max will end up safely in bed with hot dinner, welcomed home by a mom who was earlier so mad at him. Max's adventure where the Wild Things are can be understood in retrospect as the kind of wild rumpus/temper tantrum that takes kids out of their every day powerlessness to a world where they can be the king of the wild things that populate their minds. The monsters can also be understood in retrospect as what an angry parent seems like to a child: powerful, dangerous, but ultimately loving: "Please don't go. I eat you up I love you so." The complexity of the wild things in the readers' minds is prompted by just a few images; the story and its retelling suggest a casting choice that makes sense of imaginary, familiar, and powerful yet vulnerable creatures.[15]

The character is a network of disperse elements. Jonze's film brings these Wild Things to life by blending several additional sources of information. The image on screen is created partially by actors in large costumes and partially through computer-generated animation. The creatures' bodies move the way humans move, despite their very different bodies. They seem like Big Bird or sports mascots—we can almost sense the person inside. The faces do not move the way puppets or mascots move; the faces move the way computer-generated creatures move; that is to say, with as many facial muscles and expressions as humans have. Sonny Gerasimowicz, the artist who did the designs for the creatures, spoke highly of Henson, the company that did the live-action puppets for the film: "If they can get one of the most famous personalities out of a green sock with two white little balls on top—bring that to these things, we'll be good." The physical work of the actor in the suit was also important, and when they couldn't get the right physicality out of the actor in the suit for Alexander, Jonze asked Gerasimowicz to try to "act" within the suit: "I know the character already. I designed the character. . . . I think we can do it enough because the face is going to be done in post and the voice is done by Paul Dano and I wasn't the entire thing. I was like this element."[16] Although the computer anima-

tion that brought the faces to life seems like a seamless extension of the costume, the person in it, and the voice of the actor, it
is also just another "element" in the creation of character.

I am often aware of the integration network that pulls all
these elements together, despite being masked, while watching
animated films. Although the actor does not embody the character, he or she provides a voice that brings access to their celebrity.
In animated films, there are many times when the voice of the
celebrity is barely recognizable and others when it seems like the
star almost shares the screen with the graphics. Lewis Black, who
was cast as the voice of Anger in the Pixar film *Inside Out*, evokes
(perhaps only for the parents in the audience) his angry comedy
routine on *The Daily Show*. Tom Hanks and Tim Allen are present
on-screen in *Toy Story* as Woody and Buzz Lightyear; they share
a celebrity persona of honesty and integrity. Hanks and Allen are
unthreatening presences in the room of an eight-year-old. Had
the director cast Kevin Spacey, who starred in *Seven* and *Usual
Suspects* that same year, as Woody and Val Kilmer, who starred
in *Batman Forever* that year, as Buzz, no amount of quality acting
could have made those awakened dolls anything but threatening.

In *Where the Wild Things Are*, Carol, a large, impossible mon-
ster with the voice of a large man (ghosted, for many, by his role
as a damaged mafia don) is given lines that make it clear that,
in addition to being violent and angry, he is also creative, alone,
and very sad. What's wonderful about Jonze's casting is the way
the paradox of Gandolfini's character on *The Sopranos* matches
and adds to the paradox of Max's Wild Thing. Gandolfini is never
visible on-screen—the bulk of what we generally think of as "acting" (movement, staging, interacting with Max) is done by the
man in the suit and the computer graphics—but the character
seems impossibly unfinished without his voice and his ghosts.
Gandolfini is also a wonderful actor, and it is not just the ghost
of Tony Soprano that brings such richness to the role. Addition-
ally, the movie came out years after *The Sopranos* series finished,
and presumably there were many in the audience who did not
know the voice and figure of James Gandolfini as Tony Soprano.

Not all spectators will build the same character that I did while watching Gandolfini voice the words written by Spike Jonze and Dave Eggers in a story created by Sendak, in a creature designed by Gerasimowicz and constructed by Henson Studios; my experience, though, enriching my Carol with some Tony, exposed the presence of past characters and the multiple sources of information available when I build a character.

Talent

Gandolfini was a talented actor; his Tony Soprano had complexity and nuance. Talent, though, is not magic fairy dust that allows someone to play any part in any play at any time. Talent requires technique, but a technique matched to the role and to the conventions of the drama or film. The talent required to build a character in a Sophocles play involves projecting complicated poetic language through a mask, managing the stichomythia with the other character, and generating extraordinary focus and energy in a body that is mostly still. A talented actor in a drama by Arthur Miller or Tennessee Williams knows that the character is built where the secret is hid, the secret that will eventually become known in an emotional display. An actor in a George Bernard Shaw drama must be able to convey complicated rhetoric and mount strong arguments with ease. A rhetorical ability is necessary for working with Shaw or Aaron Sorkin that is less important than the perceived emotional volubility a Miller or Williams play requires. When a spectator perceives talent, he or she also perceives great casting; whether the actor is well-known or unknown, talent comes in part from the relationship between technique and role.

Some characters, no matter who the author is, seem to demand a star turn: George C. Scott, Dustin Hoffman, Brian Dennehy, and Philip Seymour Hoffman took their turns as Willy Loman; David Garrick, Kenneth Branagh, and Benedict Cumberbatch took their turns as Hamlet. These stars have talent and the technique necessary for these large, culturally important roles, but they also command attention and respect as stars. They bring importance and interpretation onstage with them. These are all stars known more for having talent than for being famous; their celebrity comes from an ability to complicate a character they become. In other words, a spectator building a character from Dustin Hoffman's performance in *The Graduate* or *Tootsie* has a multitude of conflicting stimuli that pleasurably comes together as a character at the outer edges of what makes sense. Some roles require actors who bring these multitudes with them. Francis Ford Coppola wanted to cast unknowns in his film of Mario Puzo's *The Godfather*, but he didn't think he could do that for the title role, "what actor is 60 years old and hasn't done anything?" The studio had many actors they wanted to play Vito Corleone, and Coppola and Puzo only wanted Marlon Brando. Marlon Brando, as Roach articulates, is one of those actors who "create a continuous category crisis at twenty-four frames per second (or the digitized equivalent of that analogical pace), oscillating between categories in the minds of spectators."[17]

As I argued in the last chapter about cameo parts, some characters seem written to highlight the actor's background, celebrity, and body type, while others benefit from being played by actors who are not well-known. By bringing unknowns into the world of *The Godfather*, in characters like Al Pacino's Michael Corleone and Robert Duvall's Tom Hagen, Coppola brought a paucity of information to the character-building experience of his audience. Audiences had to focus on the story and the details of how characters behaved in the circumstances in order to create a network of associations and anticipations that became Michael Corleone. Without background information about the actor to distract them, the character building depended most on the specific choices made by the actor (Duvall's choice not to laugh with the others and his resigned deep breath when Michael says that he will kill the two policemen comes to mind) and the details of the story. Of course, Pacino had the ability to make us believe he could be the straight-laced military hero at the start and also the man who orders the hit on his brother-in-law and lies to his wife about it at the end. The audience could not have made predictions about the character based on the past of an actor they did not know.

Tatiana Maslany plays many characters on *Orphan Black*, the Canadian TV show about clones. She plays Sarah, the punkish grifter; Alison, the prim housewife with a yoga mat, a pill habit, and a gun; Helena, the feral, murderous Ukrainian; Rachel, the ice-cold and razor-sharp executive; and several more. Moreover, Maslany is almost always in a scene as two or more characters, so, as one reporter put it, "she has chemistry with *herself*."[18] Sometimes the plot requires one of Maslany's characters to pretend to be one of the others, and the audience sees the work she does to make character one become character two, even though they occupy the same body:

> On more than one occasion, she plays one clone pretending to be another, exposing her own fakery in precise titrations, so that we sense the pretender's anxieties and her miscalculations. This could easily come off as a circus trick, a gimmick. And yet it doesn't: with her observant black eyes, wide smile, and an array of wigs, tics, and accents, Maslany makes herself invisible in a situation that practically demands hammy showmanship. It's a tour de force of subtlety.[19]

How can an actor make herself invisible? As I talked to friends and colleagues while working on this project, I was surprised by how many times people referred to actors they felt "disappeared" into the parts and compared this with actors they have tired of because "he always plays himself." I want to explore this language of disappearance versus self and what allows some actors to "lose themselves" and others to stage themselves. Maslany's talent comes in her ability to convey many things simultaneously — as one character or as many — but the audience can enjoy this in part because Maslany is not a known actress.

In the view of some, *Orphan Black* is not about the virtuosity of Maslany but rather about the limited roles for women on TV and in life and the need to come together, despite our (perceived) differences, to demand more freedom over our bodies and our futures. The permeability of the characters and the invisibility of the actor is what led Lili Loufbourrow of the *New York Times Magazine* to call the show a "meditation on femininity":

> By structuring the story around the clones' differences, "Orphan Black" seems to suggest that the dull sameness enforced by existing female archetypes [on TV] needs to die. Early in the first season, there is a serial killer hunting down the clones—it turns out to be Helena, the Ukrainian—who ritualistically dismembers Barbie dolls after dyeing their hair to match that of her next victim. It's a creepy touch, but one that can also be read as a metacriticism of how women are used on TV: the punishing beauty standards to which they're held, the imposed uniformity. (Need a new sitcom wife? Grab the prototype and change the hairstyle.) Our low tolerance for difference among female characters means that they will almost always be less interesting, less memorable and less beloved than their male counterparts. In this context, Helena becomes a kind of hero, slaughtering televisual conformity and constituting, in both her savagery and her warmth, a radical expansion of what women on television can be. And each character, including the criminally insane one, gets considerable attention and respect.[20]

Spectators, perhaps specifically female spectators, are hungry for the kind of cognitive workout they get with the male character paired with the "new sitcom wife": actors building characters that do the unexpected, look different (even while being played by the same actress), and widen the field of possible characters available onscreen. For Loufbourrow, good characters are interesting, memorable, and beloved, and these three adjectives also describe three different ways spectators engage with characters. Interest suggests a need to complete or make sense of the character, as if there is a mystery requiring cognitive completion. A memorable character will remain in long-term memory, available for making sense of future characters. And a beloved character evokes an emotional reaction that will draw attention and focus. "A crucial element of the esthetic experience," according to neuroscientists David Freedberg and Vittorio Gallese, "consists of the activation of embodied mechanisms encompassing the simulation of actions, emotions and corporeal sensation."[21] When casting directors, directors, and writers are more interested in the male characters and cast actors for the "wife" part based on a limited palette of acceptable body types and looks, spectators do not build the kind of complicated characters needed for this enriching esthetic experience. Maslany may bring the exact same body to each role in *Orphan Black*, but spectators attend to the conflicting, complex, and various characters possible via one actress.

Maslany makes each character interesting, memorable, and beloved in part because none of them rely on information about the actor's world or past outside of the fictional world. By disappearing as actor, Maslany stages the interchangeability of the uninteresting roles traditionally available to women on TV. The actors usually chosen to play the crime procedural scientist, tough kid, housewife, or cold female executive vary about as much from actor to actor as Maslany varies from character to character. Her disappearance has thematic value: it is part of the experience of the drama. An equally talented actor with a more visible character as an actress—Jennifer Lawrence, say, or Michelle Williams—would upstage the various characters, and we might not experience the rich thematic themes that Loufbourrow articulates. Maslany's disappearance allows spectators to remain focused on the roles and perspectives of her characters. If the actor was visible—the way it is, say, in Charlton Heston's Priam in Kenneth Branagh's *Hamlet*—or if her previous roles were visible—the way they are, say, in Robin William's Osric—we would have to keep in mind an additional perspective or presence that, in this case, would likely strain our ability to keep track of the levels of intentionality.[22] Maslany's ability to do this, to be the cipher of our experience, compels us. Articles about her and the show may talk about her "disappearing," but she remains the focus of the articles. In the *New Yorker*, Emily Nussbaum acknowledged that Maslany is not a well-known actress: "If you haven't heard of Maslany before, that's probably because she's Canadian, from Saskatchewan; her previous credits are for things like *Ginger Snaps 2*, the sequel to the cult lesbian-werewolf film (which I'd also recommend, as long as you're going Canadian)." Her past is unknown and thus doesn't compete with the many different pasts of the characters she is playing.

This seems to be a common thread among actors known for "disappearing": they are, and attempt to remain, relatively unknown as celebrities. These are rarely the actors who are found drinking coffee or filling up their gas tank "just like us" in the magazines next to the gum in the grocery store. Robert Duvall lives on a farm in Virginia and "doesn't like to attract attention to himself":

> With this impressive list [of characters played], Duvall proved his versatility but, at the same time, blended anonymously into his roles in a way that defies the usual definition of "stardom." He's never sentimental with a character. He never asks for sympathy for a character. He never tries to be "appealing" in a movie starish way. Robert Duvall is merely the character. He loses himself.[23]

The metaphor of "losing oneself" is illuminating because it suggests that there is a "self" that is separable from the actor's body, that acting is a trance whereby the "self" gets lost and a new character is channeled by the host body. The fact that this makes no sense has not stopped it from dominating the language of actors and characters. Rick Kemp points out how central metaphors of the self are to different ideas of acting: "*Many of the proclaimed differences between approaches to acting are actually differences in the types of metaphors used to describe the self and process.*"[24] Kemp's *Embodied Acting* integrates cognitive science into his approach to acting and finds that an actor like Laurence Olivier had an "essential" view of the self. For Kemp, there are "persona" actors and "transformational" actors: "The persona actor uses behavioral communicators that stay within a range that identifies his or her personality which remains more or less constant from one role to the next. The transformational actor displays a variety of behavioral communicators according to the demands of character."[25] A transformational actor will benefit from keeping distracting information about his/her personal life out of the public eye, whereas the persona actor benefits from this exposure.

One actor who is often said to disappear into his characters is Daniel Day-Lewis. Although he is famous, he is rarely seen performing his celebrity in the pages of magazines. He lives with his wife and children in County Wicklow, Ireland, and is rumored to have spent a few years working as a cobbler in Florence, Italy. We may be impressed with Day-Lewis's performance as Lincoln, but we are not moved or affected because we believe we are watching Lincoln; we know we are watching a strange trick where one become another. Bert States would call this the "self-expressive mode," in which we are "reacting to the actor's particular way of *doing* his role": "The rationale for positing such a mode of performance is that there ought to be a word, or a way of isolating, something as powerful as the pleasure we take when artistry becomes the object of our attention."[26] In Kemp's terms it might be transformational, but States attends to the spectator's interest in the spectacle of transforming as much as the product of transformation. Watching Day-Lewis as Lincoln, we are struck by the virtuosity of the actor's ability to become the character—as if we were no longer watching Lincoln or Day-Lewis but rather the pure ability to transform or disappear.

There are many contributors—author, director, costume designer, actor, set designer—but the character is built when the spectator casts the net around all these factors—including or excluding information about the actor's past. Because spectators are not distracted by stories and images of Duvall's or Day-Lewis's or Maslany's social life or past roles, they are not aware of the labor of acting either, and this is a contributing factor to the perception of talent: the seeming invisibility of the labor of acting. I do not want to downplay the contribution of talent and skill—or the designers and writers—in the creation of character but rather attend to the undertheorized network of associations required for extraordinary casting. And what this networked conception of character reveals about the perception of performance. Skill alone is not enough. Even Maslany or Day-Lewis could not play any part. This is the kind of statement that gets me into trouble: many people want to believe that the right skill, technique, and art can transform any actor into any character. Daniel Day-Lewis's choices to remain out of celebrity magazines and his tremendous talent and skill, does not actually render him invisible, a kind of disembodied talent force. For the 2013 White House Correspondent's Dinner, Obama's White House created a video called Steven Spielberg's "Obama," which featured Spielberg talking about casting for his movie-version of the Obama presidency.[27] The right actor to play Obama, he decides, is Daniel Day-Lewis; "he becomes his characters." During the video, Obama is interviewed as Day-Lewis playing Obama, as if Day-Lewis was such a transformational actor that he could, actually transform. Obama (as Day-Lewis playing Obama) says, "Was it hard playing Obama? I'll be honest, it was. This accent took awhile" then we watch Obama practicing in front of a dressing room mirror: "Hello, Ohio! Hello, Ohio." The humor comes from the recognition of just how ridiculous this casting choice is. Even Daniel Day-Lewis can't play any part. What an attention to casting reveals is that there are physical requirements to this ability.

Bodies that Matter

Perhaps part of what we perceive as talent in an actor is his or her ability to work with the body he or she brings to the role. In her *Four Lectures on Shakespeare*, Ellen Terry discusses the distance between Sarah Siddons's impression of Lady Macbeth and the impression her performance made on an audience member. Siddons, according to Terry, thought Lady Macbeth was "fair, feminine, nay perhaps even fragile," but a spectator described Siddons' Lady M as an "exultant savage."[28] Terry determines that

> It is not always possible for us players to portray characters on the stage exactly as we see them in imagination. Mrs. Siddons may have realized that her physical appearance alone—her aquiline nose, her raven hair, her flashing eyes, her commanding figure—was against her portraying a fair, feminine, "nay perhaps even fragile" Lady Macbeth. It is no use an actress wasting her nervous energy on a battle with her physical attributes. She had much better find a way of employing them as allies.[29]

Siddons's physical attributes were an inescapable part of what she brought onstage for each character. Moreover, these attributes had been selected as salient by a public interested in just such a figure. Celebrities, those whom Roach might define as having It, exist in relationship to a social/cultural environment that needs what those particular bodies bring: "Perhaps then, . . . actors with It are not merely there *for* us; they are there *instead* of us—there to live the sort of lives we can imagine and desire but for which we lack the courage, the gift, or the luck—in short, the It—to live for ourselves. In that sense, we are also there for them."[30] Siddons could often make her "raven hair, her flashing eyes, her commanding figure" allies because she lived in a time and place where her particular combination of the maternal and the sexual was powerful.

Carrie Fisher, the iconic princess from the original Star Wars franchise, was asked to lose thirty-five pounds before she could return to her role as Princess Leia for Episode VII. As she said in an interview with *Good Housekeeping*: "They don't want to hire all of me—only about three quarters. I'm in a business where the only thing that matters is weight and appearance. That is so messed up. They might as well say get younger, because that's how easy it is."[31] Of course, she also received attention from fans and the media about whether or not she had plastic surgery.[32] As Sue Bell put it in a post for midlifeexpress.com, "Would it really have been too much for audiences to cope with an older (and fatter) Princess Leia? Shouldn't midlife take its natural course? Does Leia have to retain a semblance of youth for people to care about her character? And how can a 59-year-old face pulled taut and tight like a newborn be more convincing to audiences than the wrinkled skin and extra pounds of a late middle-aged woman?"[33] Princess Leia wasn't allowed to gain a few pounds and age a few years after defeating the Galactic Empire, and Leslie Jones couldn't find a dress designer for the premiere of *Ghostbusters* (2016).[34] Some bodies do not disappear into a role, and while weight might help convey conviviality or vulnerability in a man (John Goodman, John Candy, James Gandolfini), it tends to mark women as villains or jokes (Kathy Bates, Melissa McCarthy). If Maslany gained Fisher's thirty-five pounds, she would not have "disappeared" into her various clone characters.

In contemporary American society, few things mark a body as visibly as race. Often scholars who write about casting discuss questions of race. In fact, Angela Pao argues that the nontraditional casting that has happened since the civil rights era changed how we viewed casting:

> The very idea of a casting schema as a semantic field or an interpretive register for a dramatic text emerged only when the race or ethnicity of the actor became a relevant factor. The casting of dramatic roles, heretofore relegated to the semiotic cellars of theatrical convention or mimetic correspondence, became elevated to the status of an expressive language of the stage.[35]

While casting has always controlled interpretation, the visibility of these "theatrical conventions" increases when the standards of a white male-centered perspective are challenged. For Pao, nontraditional casting opens up a space between character and actor, "prompting the spectator to exercise new modes of perception and learn new protocols of reception."[36] If the body playing the part matches what the spectator assumes it should be (a younger, thinner Carrie Fisher), then perhaps it is possible to fail to notice the modes of perception that integrated size and race into character building. If the body playing the part does not match the presumed race of the character—Lin-Manuel Miranda as Alexander Hamilton, for example—spectators learn protocols of reception that question the central importance, the normality, the invisibility of white bodies.

The power of race in this society marks some bodies, as August Wilson argued in his famous 1996 debate with Robert Brustein on the problems with "color-blind casting." Wilson, a self-described "race man," argued against color-blind casting because it "assaults" African Americans by denying their unique past. Brustein responded that Wilson's position was tantamount to "subsidized separatism."[37] Brandi Wilkins Catanese's book on black performance, *The Problem of the Color [blind]*, insightfully argues against both of their positions, shifting the focus to the institutional racism that makes color-blind casting the way to give black actors access to the "superior" high art of white authors and recuperating it as a site of possible transgression, which she prefers to transcendence. Asking (usually people of color) to "transcend" race, Catanese points out, is often another way of asking them to "get over it." On the other hand, the "cultural and aesthetic practices that push at these very finite demarcations of the acceptable and unacceptable, the just and the unjust, enable us to imagine and then create alternatives for people whose concerns would otherwise be dismissed through the silencing tyranny of color blindness."[38] She argues,

> In defiance of both Wilson's dogma about authentic blackness and Brustein's weariness with "indictment and complaint," color-blind casting may contribute to the multivalence of black subjectivity by insisting upon the relevance of black bodies and the intertext of black culture to a wider variety of narratives than are currently staged. . . . The dialogue between the culture of the play and the culture of the contemporary world in which audiences are situated underscores color-blind casting's function as one vehicle among many for expanding how we understand blackness and its value.[39]

Wilkins then analyzes a high-profile example of color-blind casting, Denzel Washington in *The Pelican Brief* (1993), and finds Washington's race glaringly visible when set in relationship with co-star Julia Roberts' race.

As Catanese points out, the film, based on John Grisham's novel, does not explicitly alter the race of Washington's character and wants to create a "color-blind space."[40] However, the "inherent racialization of aesthetics" means that the sexual attraction between the two main characters must be carefully sidestepped because of the visibility of Washington's blackness and Roberts's whiteness. The scene in the film that comes closest to staging attraction between them "alternates between exploiting the cultural celebrity of the actors and supporting the narrative. Washington is repeatedly shot in close-ups, giving the audience time to savor his good looks, and Roberts is shown in three-quarter body shots, keeping her a bit more distant from viewers."[41] Catanese finds in the film and in reports from the author, the director, and the star incredible consciousness about the choices made in light of the film's historical and cultural context. Washington certainly was not blind to his own race or how it would be read as he thought about his acting choices. Fresh from his Oscar win for *Training Day* in 2002, Washington's performance in *The Pelican Brief*, according to Catanese, proves that race is almost always a powerful part of performance.

In 2015 and 2016—particularly in the lead-up to the 2016 Oscars, many people in the media discussed questions of race and casting. In February 2015, when *Hamilton* opened at The Public Theatre in New York, reviews and interest exploded. Even in the first review, Ben Brantley quipped that the show "has become the most fashionable (and unobtainable) ticket in town."[42] Reviewers wrote of the thematic impact of the casting, in which the Founding Fathers are played by nonwhites: "The casting of multicultural actors in these historical roles accentuates the parallels between the revolutionary aims of the characters and the ongoing struggle to extend this grand democratic project to all people."[43] Casting a Latino as Alexander Hamilton and an

African American as Aaron Burr does not confuse our historical recollection of the character, nor does it ask that we "look
past" the race of the actors. The casting creates new characters in
a network of history, future, bodies, and colors. In an interview
with Howard Sherman, Lin-Manuel Miranda, the creator and
MacArthur genius behind *Hamilton*, said that he is not yet sure
how he will specify casting when the acting edition of the show
is published and it is made available for production at schools
across the country,[44] but he notes that the London cast will be
as diverse as the current show, adding that "there are going to be
even more opportunities for southeast Asian and Asian and communities of color within Europe that should be represented on
stage in that level of production."[45] Casting, for him, is not about
mimesis, and it's not about bestowing opportunities on talented
performers; it's about how the racial and ethnic makeup of the
performers speaks with and through the story of the birth of democracy. Without representing onstage the "young, scrappy, and
hungry" people who might rebuild a democracy now, *Hamilton*
isn't *Hamilton*.

In June 2015, the National Asian American Theater Company
did a production of *Awake and Sing!* at The Public Theatre with
a cast of Asian Americans (from Korean, Chinese, Indian, Japa-
nese, Sri Lankan, and Filipino descent). Reviewing it for the *New
York Times*, Laura Collins-Hughes did not focus on the casting
choices: "What might seem the most noteworthy thing about
this staging—that these are Asian-American actors playing Jewish American characters—is, in practice, unremarkable. It's a
classic American story, and that means that it belongs to all of
us."[46] While this may be true, a story from a similar historical period about a nonwhite American family is unlikely to be considered a "classic" and be unmarked by racial concerns the way this
story is.[47] Further, it is the casting choice of the play that brought
it to the Public; The Public is unlikely to be interested in a revival
of a Clifford Odets play. Mia Katigbak, founder of the National Asian American Theater Company, specifically mentioned her
hope that such a performance might expand the opportunities

for Asian Americans in TV and film: "If people can buy us as a Jewish-American family in the 1930s, maybe they'll look at us differently the next time."[48]

The more contentious fall of 2015 brought two productions under fire for casting against the intentions of the author—although these playwrights were alive to voice their concerns. Katori Hall's *The Mountaintop*, about a conversation between Dr. Martin Luther King and a hotel maid, was produced at Kent State University with a white actor playing Dr. King. Hall later wrote in an article for *Root* about her anger: "While it is true that I never designated in the play text that King and Camae be played by black actors, reading comprehension and good-old scene analysis would lead any director to cast black or darker-complexioned actors." In addition to the historical knowledge spectators bring to the production about the race of Dr. King—and the importance of his race—the text of the play explicitly mentions the "chocolate" skin color of Dr. King. Hall has now added a clause to her licensing agreement to affirm the dramaturgical and ideological good sense of casting an African American actor to play Dr. King.[49] My support for Hall's position is not that actors can never take on a role written for another race, nor is it an argument about the paucity of roles for actors of color and thus roles written for actors of color should be given to actors of color. My argument is that to deny the importance of the actor's skin color in casting a role like Dr. King is to deny the importance of the character's skin color and that does dramaturgical and ideological harm.

While Hall did not find out about the casting decisions at Kent State until after the performance had closed, Lloyd Suh discovered that two white actors and a mixed-race performer had been cast to play the Indians in his play *Jesus in India* at Clarion University in Pennsylvania before the production opened and was able to cancel it. In an essay for *American Theatre*, Diep Tran insisted that author's intent had to come before other considerations in casting. Further, Tran argued that "now ain't the time for white tears," which he defines as "that unfortunate phenomenon that sees any questioning of long-standing white privilege, in this case the right to play any role of any ethnicity, as an inequity on par with institutional racism, as if the playing field were level."[50] The problem for me is not opportunities on either side but rather the lack of insight into what pieces of information about the actor's body are relevant in the portrayal of the character by the actor and then built by the spectator. It is not the talent of the actor playing Dr. King or the characters in Suh's play that matter, it is the idea that white skin is neutral and provides an all-access pass to all characters, all performances. A spectator building that particular Dr. King—a Dr. King with a white body—comes to see race as something you can visit or mimic or perform. Such an idea mocks the very struggles Dr. King died for and Hall's play explores. White skin in America is privilege; to insist that acting can perform away that privilege is insulting. While I may not agree with everything August Wilson espouses in his powerful (and no less timely) 1996 Theatre Communications Group address, recognition of difference is critical for art:

> We can meet on the common ground of theater as a field of work and endeavor. But we cannot meet on the common ground of experience. Where is the common ground in the horrifics of lynching? Where is the common ground in the maim of a policeman's bullet? Where is the common ground in the hull of a slave ship and the deck of a slave ship with its refreshments of air and expanse? We will not be denied our history.[51]

We must understand how spectators—all of us—build characters in order to see and honor what is there.

In September 2015, Viola Davis won an Emmy for her portrayal of a lawyer on How to Get Away with Murder. In her acceptance speech, she spoke of the need for opportunity: "The only thing that separates women of color from anyone else is opportunity. You cannot win an Emmy for roles that are simply not there." She did not talk about being cast in more roles written for white actors but rather about having more writers write parts that redefine "what it means to be beautiful, to be sexy, to be a leading woman. To be black." For Davis, it's not the opportunity to play Leonardo DiCaprio's love interest that is the problem; it's the opportunity for a wider variety of stories told by a wider variety of bodies.

In response to the Oscars So White controversy, the *New York Times* ran a series of interviews with Hollywood actors, directors, and producers called "What It's Really Like to Work in Hollywood* (*If You're Not a Straight White Man)." Actress Theyonah Parris talked about finding a new way of taking on a role in a nontraditionally cast play:

> I looked at actresses who were white doing these classics and, like, O.K., this is how it's supposed to be. We were doing Chekhov; I was playing Yelena. Liesl Tommy [a black South African woman who was guest directing at Juilliard] called me on everything. At the time, I did not understand what she was saying: Use yourself. Yelena [was] still a white woman in my head. As opposed to [now], Yelena is a black woman who comes with the life experience that I can draw from.[52]

Catanese writes about a similar experience playing Rosalind in *As You Like It*, when she realized that she had to respond to lines about the "white hand of Rosalind" without the "same skin color Shakespeare imagined for her."[53] Instead of hoping her audience would not respond to the "dissonance between words and body," she capitalized on the disconnect:

> when he uttered the fateful line, I snuck a peek at my brown hand in momentary confusion, then continued to nod encouragingly. The audience laughed, and our scene was a success. I couldn't not acknowledge the material specificity of my body in that moment of performance, but I didn't quite know what to do, so I took it as my responsibility to demonstrate my awareness of my nonnormative performing body.[54]

These kinds of transgressions are possible and productive. These kinds of "bad manners" (Catanese's seductive term) increase insight. These kinds of transgressions, according to Ayanna Thompson, are what Shakespeare in America has always afforded.

There's a reason why Shakespeare is so often the site of "nontraditional" casting. In her book *Passing Strange*, Thompson shows "how well and how comfortably Shakespeare and race fit together in American imagination." Thompson focuses on "how and why instability is the nature of the relationship between Shakespeare and race in American popular culture."[55] She insists that "both the artistry and the ideology" should be examined when thinking about casting and Shakespeare, noting that "color-blind" casting in Shakespeare is often used to support the argument of Shakespeare's universality, as if Shakespeare is so powerful that spectators can see differently within his world. Others insist that there is no such thing as a play freed from history, but

> both sides assume that race does not always exist in performance. The universalist/non-naturalist argument assumes that whiteness is normative and, therefore, not raced. The cultural-specifist/naturalist argument is often so focused on actors of color that it neglects race in/as performance *in terms of whiteness itself.*[56]

Shakespeare may satisfy a desire to find a world where we can pretend that race and performance are not always intimately related, but performance of character onstage and off is always connected to race and social position.

White performers in America are given a kind of VIP pass to enter whatever character-door they want to because white America is not always presumed to be carrying its race around. In fact, the erasure of race is a large part of why white celebrities are seen as providing a surrogate; in Roach's sense, he or she is there for us, both better and also incomplete. The "nude" in the crayon box, a white actor provides the most people with the most potential access and identification—and without that ease of travel, how

could he or she have "It"? In *Performing Glam Rock,* Philip Auslander argues that the persona of rock stars is an integral part of
the reception of their music, particularly in glam rock, which was
"defined primarily by the performers' appearances and personae,
the poses they struck rather than the music they played."[57] Rock
stars create a persona with multiple layers of information that
informs our experience of their music. Auslander's analysis of
David Bowie, for example, puts his various personae in the contexts of glam rock's reaction to the hippie counterculture, "rock
culture's traditional heterosexual imperative,"[58] and the radical
presentation of a fluid queer identity: "Bowie's concert performances of Ziggy Stardust were the culmination of the three
intertwined tendencies I have been discussing: his continual
challenges to rock's ideology of authenticity, his desire to theatricalize rock performance, and his engagement in complex representations of gender and sexuality."[59] David Bowie called attention to his persona by changing costumes and highlighting the
theatricality; he passed seamlessly from one identity to the next
where others may have gotten stuck.

African American performers, on the other hand, are often
stopped at the border of potential transgressive performances. "Bitches ain't shit," from Dr. Dre's debut album, *The Chronic*
(1992), tells a story of friendship and betrayal with the various
singers' stories returning to the rat-a-tat chorus of: "Bitches ain't
shit but hoes and tricks / Lick on these nuts and suck the dick
/ Get the fuck out after you're done / And I hops in my ride to
make a quick run."[60] Dr. Dre and collaborators Snoop Dog, Daz,
and Kurupt describe variations of the troublesome eponymous
"bitches." The album and the song were immediately held up as
examples of the horrors of misogyny in rap culture.[61] Nelson
Havelock of *Rolling Stone* said of the album as a whole that "cops
and other folks get wasted ('Dem punk mutha-fuckas in black and
white ain't the only muthafuckas I gots ta fight') in a sometimes
frightening amalgam of inner-city street games that includes
misogynist sexual politics and violent revenge scenarios."[62] Billboard's "Classic Track-By-Track Review," published twenty years

after the album came out, noted that "the misogyny is ugly and thick, even for a rap record."[63] In an editorial in the *New York Times*, Brent Staples noted that "these lyrics [of power, violence, and misogyny] go out to an audience of young black men who are being murdered at five times the national average."[64] He viewed the problem that the cultural ideology embodied in gangsta rap has created as the way it "determines how we see them, how they see themselves and, to a large extent, what they aspire to become."[65] The trouble, as Jon Pareles notes about *Dogg Food*, a later album put out by Death Row Records, is that

> The Death Row formula makes gangster life seem like a swank men's club. It's the Playboy Philosophy plus weapons: bond with the boys, rake in the case, take the women as spoils. The rude language helps the album appeal to nose-thumbing adolescent sensibilities and will draw the condemnations it's asking for, even as its sleaziness boosts sales. But what really makes "Dogg Food" such a commercial proposition is the escape—simultaneously virile and pampered—promised in the music.[66]

The performers on the album and those who listen in the car or at home are all promised an escape to the world where a gat and a bitch-slap can solve most problems. The music creates a character for Dr. Dre and the others to play and gives listeners access to that character's perspective.

Even, perhaps, women. While I am not likely to be found singing "Bitches Ain't Shit" in the shower, it always slightly troubled me that my favorite music to work out to requires me to sing lyrics such as "so we start lookin' for the bitches with the big butt, like her, but she keeps crying 'I got a boyfriend' bitch stop lying! Dumb ass hooker aint nothin' but a dyke." This song, "Gangsta Gangsta" by N.W.A., from their seminal album of 1988, *Straight Outta Compton*, tells the tale of police lulling, assault, and female intimidation, if not rape. Its protagonist proclaims himself "the type of nigga that's built to last," which is not the first or the last time I notice that the song is definitely not written from my point of view; I am neither. The distance between my perspective and the perspective of the singer is part of my joy, part of the power of my experience of the song. Just as most black men in America are decidedly not "built to last," my lack of connection to what I was singing actually created the power in the leap into imagining myself as a powerful outlaw, confident that any threat could be met with a stronger counterthreat. Put another way, based on the casting protocols Pao refers to in the "semiotic cellars of theatrical convention or mimetic,"[67] I would be cast as the "dumb ass hooker," not the n-word "built to last." Onstage, my whiteness and my feminine characteristics would cause the audience to question the very thing I question: how can I possibly take on the perspective of one when I am so clearly the other? Unless the protocols of casting are not what we think they are.

The insistence that gangsta rappers created exaggerated characters for popular consumption did not do much to quell the response to the music. Dr. Dre looks like a gangster (and tabloid information gives us background information that portrays the actor behind the character as a violent misogynist[68]) and the lines he speaks in songs like "Bitches Ain't Shit" confirm this interpretation. When, however, Ben Folds covered the song in 2005, the song received a slightly different reception. This is not to say that it wasn't perceived as misogynist: during a live performance, Folds explained that "It's funny because I didn't write the lyrics to this thing and I've almost been beaten up a couple of times over this. Once by a kind of uptight hippie woman who said it was demeaning to women and I was like: 'Really? I guess I could read that between the lines.'"[69] The audience laughs at his sarcasm, and the humor assures the room that no offense is meant. He is not a danger; he gets the joke. He refers the woman to the "lyrics department," which is Dr. Dre. He goes on to say that he thinks the story in the song is very sad and every story has two sides and "this is the sad side; Dre told it like it was a joke and, um, this isn't a joke, it's fucking serious." The audience is in it with him, singing along, shouting out "so true!" after the first "bitches ain't shit." The artsy white man at the piano can make it funny while making it sad, and the lyrics support both interpretations; the casting is what makes the difference.

There are salient differences in the performance, of course. Ben Folds sitting at a piano evokes an old-fashioned crooner or lounge act. The recording on Dr. Dre's album (the only performance I can find) is three men singing together about different people. We can only imagine the song sung by the tough-looking black man on the album cover who, along with his crew, has worked very hard to maintain an authentic streets and gang authority. The simplistic performance analysis this creates is that Dr. Dre is a vicious misogynist, and Ben Folds is an ironic performance artist. While I am not going to argue about what may or may not be true about the individual artists, I am struck by how our casting of the lyrics can bring an experience of sadness to one performance and a callous humor to the other. Yet the more I watched performances of Ben Folds singing this song at concerts, the more I felt that his innocuous white guy performance masked a troubling experience. The cackles and singing from the audiences suggest that they are hailed by the song, welcomed in, and engaged to be part of it. And they like it. They don't seem to be saddened by the song; they seemed to be delighted to be able to laugh at the sad situation. Further, while it seems clear that Folds is trespassing into Dre's gangsta character in order to point out that the song is both sad and funny, he is also performing the all-access pass granted him by his whiteness and inviting the audience to join him.

Even I, a white female, feel impelled to join him, to sing along about how "bitches ain't shit," despite the likelihood that if the situation were to be cast, I would not get to portray Folds or Dre but perhaps one of the various "bitches." Yet this is not how I cast myself in this moment; singing along, I take on the position of the powerful, the angry, the sad, the person aggrieved by "bitches." Contemporary culture divides characters by gender primarily. Before we learn race, age, or other identifying markers, we are taught gender—which is usually presumed to be equal to sex. As Judith Butler might explain, this is our first performance mandate. This does not mean it will always be this way or that it has been this way forever. While talking about how to trick the citizenry into begging Richard of Gloucester to be king, in Shakespeare's *Richard III*, Buckingham instructs Richard in how to play the part of the coy, unwilling, candidate: "Play the maid's part, still answer nay, and take it" (3.7.51). Listening with twenty-first-century ears, I hear a reference to women saying no to sex but meaning yes. But to Shakespearean ears, the "maid's part" would have been played by a boy, an indentured apprentice who played the maid's parts in the plays and had to accept whatever demands were placed on him. Powerless boys in the position of saying no but taking it are cast as maids because of their age and powerlessness, not because of their penis.[70]

This kind of strategic miscasting, or counter casting, opens up what is perceived as possible. When the body of the actor shows through, when it isn't what was expected, the spectators must consider the nature of their expectations. Marjorie Garber argues that there is cultural power in the counter casting involved in cross-dressing: "The transvestite in this scenario is both terrifying and seductive precisely because s/he incarnates and emblematizes the disruptive element that intervenes, signaling not just another category crisis, but—much more disquietingly—a crisis of 'category' itself."[71] Garber points out how the boy player becomes linked to the monstrous; in *A Midsummer Night's Dream*, when Bottom explains how he could play the girl's part, he promises, "I'll speak in a monstrous little voice." The boy player, the "provoker of category crises, a destabilizer of binarisms,"[72] is the monstrous hybrid of two categories, proving by his monstrosity the importance of their difference. This crisis of category is my primary interest: how do we use theatre and the casting and miscasting it calls for to keep continual pressure on our categorical commitments? When, as a society, we point to the kinds of "miscasting" involved in "color-blind casting" or cross-gender casting, we illuminate what we perceived as normative and display an interest in questioning that categorization.

CHAPTER 3

MULTICASTING
The Dispersed Character

In the previous chapter, I focused on the visibility of the actor's body and the idea that some actors seem to "disappear" into a role. These are moments when casting is particularly visible, when we see the actor and the character both together and apart and the question arises: Why this actor for this part? Mostly, spectators presume mimetic matching or a meritocratic assessment of acting quality. The presumption that casting comes from matching types and finding talent masks the creative composing done when the spectator brings her associations to a particular actor in a particular part. No actor's portrayal of a character is independent of the network of mental spaces within the spectator that makes up his or her understanding of the actor and of character (the physical type of the actor, including race, gender, size, and age; the lines of dialogue spoken by the character; and the ghosts of other characters and actors). Tatiana Maslany is able to "disappear" into her roles as the many clones on *Orphan Black* partially because of her talent and also because her lack of celebrity status and her thin, white body grants her more movement than Leslie Jones's larger black body. The bodies of the actors contribute to the characters built.

These bodies—which spectators assess in a particular cultural and historical moment—are not independent of the performance context within which the spectator finds them. In other words, no actor's portrayal of character is independent of other choices made by the creative team: costumes, staging, lighting, camera angles, and many other factors can shift how an audience perceives a character. One relevant factor in how spectators build characters is the casting of the other characters; the character built by the spectator for Romeo will depend on the actor selected to play Juliet. Actors are not independent of the cast or ecosystem within which they perform. In this chapter, I examine performances that alter the ecosystem in such a way as to impact the characters built by the spectators. I start with a strange example of a casting choice—the depiction of Mary in Michelangelo's *Pietá*—to extend the idea of "casting" to other artistic representations. To support this extension, I will return to the idea of distributed cognition introduced in the first chapter. I then look at how characters and casting interact when characters are played by more than one actor or when an actor plays more than one character.

In the dark hallway of the Vatican, surrounded by visitors and guards, is Michelangelo's *Pietá*.[1] Seeing it is theatrical. You are always in an audience as tour guides and docents narrate and the sculpture seems to unfold and transform as you watch it. Mary holds her dead son, limp and sprawled across her lap. She is not keening but rather looking down on him with a beautiful sadness. The fingers of her right hand make an impression in the flesh under his right arm almost like the folds of her dress; this is the dead weight of an adult man. When art historian Giorgio Vasari saw the statue in 1550, he wrote:

> The rarest artist could add nothing to its design and grace, or finish the marble with such polish and art, for it displays the utmost limits of sculpture. Among its beauties are the divine draperies, the foreshortening of the dead Christ and the beauty of the limbs with the muscles, veins, sinews, while no better presentation of a corpse was ever made. The sweet air of the head and the harmonious join-

ing of the arms and legs to the torso, with the pulses and veins, are marvelous, and it is a miracle that a once shapeless stone should assume a form that Nature with difficulty produces in flesh.[2]

Nature, though, would have aged Mary thirty years and in flesh she would not have the size capable of holding his dead weight in her lap.

Michelangelo strategically miscast his Mary. The folds of the robe mask her size at first, but this Mary has enough room in her lap to dwarf the man. There are clearly practical reasons for this, as the sculpture could not support the weight of a second Mary-sized adult without a larger base. But the size differential evokes the mother-and-child dyads of Mary and the baby Jesus; images we are all familiar with. The beautiful face, so clearly shown in the statue (more beautiful, in fact, than that of Jesus) is one of a young woman who is the right age to have a baby, not a 32-year-old son. Some art historians suggest that this is because she is without sin and thus has not been marked by the ravages of age. This seems like a proper reading, but it does not address the phenomenological experience of viewing the image. What we see held together in front of us are two periods of time: Mary as a young mother holding her child and Jesus as a grown man dead in his mother's lap. By conflating these two time periods, Michelangelo telescopes the time of the hope of the beatific young mother and the devastation of a mother holding her dead son. Mary is miscast, but the character is built in relation to the pose, the story.

Michelangelo casts the young Mary in a scene with the old Jesus and poses them to evoke the young Jesus. Both stories happen at once: Jesus as an adult goes back to his young mother's lap to die. Mary as a young mother is famously "without sin"; she has done nothing to be with this child. The baby Jesus has done nothing yet; paintings of the child add the golden aura to presage future greatness. The adult son has done many things and is now dead. In the *Pietá*, Mary is simultaneously holding the baby who has done nothing and the adult son who has done things but retains the innocence of the infant in her arms. This becomes moving even to a secular spectator because any man dead on his mother's lap will evoke the innocence of the infant that belongs there, and any mother holding a baby is secretly terrified that one day she will hold her dead son in her lap. Michelangelo, I have to believe, could easily have sculpted a beautiful 50-year-old woman, but by casting her as the young mother, he is running two stories at once and the image is twice as heartbreaking. The experience of the *Pietá* comes from a casting choice that runs counter to realism but generates the nonsensical truth in the grieving mother image. The character comes from the relationship—at two points in time—and the spectator makes sense of this through an embodied engagement with the art.

If thinking was a process of translating semiotic information into a reading or an answer, Michelangelo's Mary would make no sense. As I look at the statue, the muscles of my fingers twitch where her fingers pucker the skin of her son. I feel the grief, the weight, and I remember other images of this dyad. The environment of the Vatican, the echoing voices off the walls, the guards, and the high ceilings inform my interaction with the sculpture. The size requires me to look up to see her face looking down at him, placing the angle of my head in position to receive the love and grief she bestows. Studies have shown that the state of the body informs interpretation. D. A. Havas and colleagues asked people to hold a pencil in their mouths, either with only their teeth or only their lips, and then to answer questions about emotionally positive or negative events. Though this awkward posturing of subjects' faces into smiles or frowns was entirely artificial and independent of endogenous emotional states, the physical position prompted the correlated emotional state. Asked to read sad sentences or happy sentences, subjects responded faster—meaning they comprehended the sentence faster—when the sentence matched the artificially generated facial expression. Frowning makes me see sad faster. This suggests that looking up at a sculpture will prompt a different reaction than looking down. Engaging with the *Pietá* means interacting with loss, with impossible grace, and with a mortal god as a dead child. This is not a semiotic reading of Mary's character independent of the environment. Spectators respond to Michelangelo's youthful cast of Mary by entering the dyad differently: the character is no longer located exclusively in Mary but is enacted in the entire experience of seeing the sculpture.

Distributed Cognition and Character Breakdown

Studies like the one with the pencil forcing a smile or frown have shown pretty clearly that thinking is something that involves the whole organism, not just the brain. How my mouth is shaped, the texture or warmth of something placed in my hand, will alter what and how I think about that thing.[3] Cognition is something that takes place in an organism embedded in an environment. The prop table organizes what the actor needs so that between scenes he or she does not need to look at the table, remember what he or she needs for the next scene, and search for those objects. The stage manager marks the paper on the table so the prop goes in the same place every night, often tracing the edge so the hammer goes where the hammer silhouette is. In this case, the actor reaching for the hammer before running on stage is an example of embodied and distributed cognition. We use prompts in our environment to guide our actions in the moment. We can take advantage of this—as the stage manager does—and alter our environment to support the offloading of cognitive tasks. David Kirsh and Paul Maglio call this "epistemic action" as opposed to "pragmatic action." They define epistemic action as actions that we take "to change the world in order to simplify the problem-solving task." In contrast, pragmatic actions are the things we do to bring us "physically closer to a goal."[4] For Kirsh and Maglio, epistemic actions might not aid movement but aids cognition, like arranging the groceries before bagging them or keeping track of numbers on our hands. We create tight feedback loops between our actions and the world they act on and with, so we can operate quickly and efficiently. Thinking is what happens between agents and the tools in their environment.

This shift to a situated view of cognition is an idea of such magnitude that it requires new language and a plethora of new terms. The term "situated cognition" has been used to encompass terms such as "embodiment, enactivism, distributed cognition, and the extended mind." Scientists and philosophers use these words to understand and articulate the complex, dynamic nature of cognition.[5] These thinkers commit to the embodiment of cognition and perceive some degree to which cognition exploits the "structure in the natural and social environments."[6] All argue for a rethinking of the way cognition transcends the boundaries that are assumed to exist between organisms. Not all who argue for the existence of situated cognition think alike; some make much stronger commitments and claims than others. Debates about when and where situated cognition happens will likely continue for some time to come. For theater and performance scholars, however, the core of the idea is what is important. For example, Evelyn Tribble extends the cognitive anthropological work of Edwin Hutchins and the cognitive theories of Andy Clark, among others, to imagine Shakespeare's Globe as a site of distributed cognition, where the cognitive load of the event is spread over and through the people, the environment, and the system.[7] To do the work of *Hamlet*, for example, required thinking with the tiring house doors; the rhythm of the poetry; the entrances and exit maps backstage; and the casting of the clown, the apprentice, and Burbage.

Persuading those in the arts and humanities that they are basing their theories on outdated assumptions about how the mind works will not be easy. Because scholars are taught to believe in deep specialization—that gaining prestige is knowing the very most about the very least—many in the arts and humanities do not think it is necessary to check their theories against new research in other fields of study. While F. Elizabeth Hart and Bruce McConachie have made powerful arguments against work that presumes a disembodied brain with modular, computer-like regions for things like language and emotion, no one wants the theoretical rug pulled out from under them.[8] Telling people for whom cinema is fundamentally about the gaze and the fetish or those who believe that literature is best understood as a symptom of a historical/cultural problem that their fundamental understanding of their field is incorrect or inadequate does not make one popular.

There are, however, exciting examples of scholars who are demonstrating the potential of this interdisciplinary turn. In a recent essay, Barbara Dancygier, a literary scholar and cognitive linguist, turns to the multimodality of stage language, arguing that props can work as dramatic anchors, holding parts of the story or meaning in their presence:

> Dramatic anchors have a dual function, and they are both material anchors (though only to the ongoing conceptualization of the play's meaning) and narrative anchors, as they contribute to the understanding of the story. They do materially participate in the performance, but they also guide the viewer in constructing the meaning of the play.[9]

For Dancygier, the tortoise that spends the entire length of Tom Stoppard's *Arcadia* (1993) walking around the table, eating scraps, and just being a tortoise is one such dramatic anchor. The play takes place in one location and two time periods, so the characters of 1809 and 1989 both leave props on and pick props up from the table; and, as Stoppard says in his stage directions, "where an object in one scene would be an anachronism in another (say a coffee mug) it is simply deemed to have become invisible."[10] Characters from both time periods, however, interact with the tortoise, connecting the two worlds in the minds of the spectators, through an apple:

> Early in the play, at the end of a scene, a character in 1809 leaves an apple on the table, and at the beginning of the next scene a charac-

ter in the other period picks it up and cuts out a slice to feed it to the tortoise. The piece of fruit thus becomes a material "connective tissue" linking the past and the present into one story.[11]

During *Arcadia*'s few hours' traffic of the stage, the characters place objects on the table (books, papers, "an old fashioned theodolite") that provide tools for their intellectual work, staging for the audience the situated nature of their cognitive tasks. Spectators also take advantage of the tools on the table to make sense of characters located in two different time periods but one common location. The tortoise and the apple further the plots in two different time periods and serve as a clue for the spectators that time must operate differently here. The characters of Gus Coverly (from 1989) and Augustus Coverly (from 1809) are both played by the same actor, connecting that character to the other living creatures that cross through the times and ecosystems of the play. In this way, the casting illuminates not something about the character but about the play: this is a world where time and place are folded and intellectual inquiry requires epistemic action.

A performance—a movie, a play, or a TV show—is what John Sutton and Evelyn Tribble refer to, following Edwin Hutchins, as a cognitive ecology:

> Cognitive ecologies are the multidimensional contexts in which we remember, feel, think, sense, communicate, imagine, and act, often collaboratively, on the fly, and in rich ongoing interaction with our environments. . . . The idea is not that the isolated, unsullied individual first provides us with the gold standard for a cognitive agent, and that mind is then projected outward into the ecological system: but that from the start (historically and developmentally) remembering, attending, intending, and acting are distributed, co-constructed, system-level activities.[12]

An audience member must build the character of Juliet based on the information provided by the casting of Romeo. I do not mean the two actors must have "chemistry"; I mean that spectators take into consideration the other characters/actors in the narrative world. We do not "read" characters one at a time like some kind of semiotic processing machine. Romeo and Juliet are bad examples, perhaps, because the unexplained hatred between the Montagues and the Capulets has often been explained by casting the families as different races. The point is that spectators do not make sense of characters in isolation. The casting of Sam Shepard as the ghost of King Hamlet in Michael Almereyda's *Hamlet* gained meaning and consequence because he was cast against Ethan Hawke as Hamlet:

> With Shepard as the dead father returning to seek revenge from his dawdling son, there is an added pathos to Shepard's/Ghost's disappointment and Hawke's/Hamlet's anxiety about revenge: this is probably not the first time Shepard/Ghost has found his son Hawke/Hamlet lacking in strength, action or integrity. When Shepard first appears to Hawke, he charges him, intimidates him and silences him. Sam Shepard is the strong cowboy to Hawke's disaffected Gen X intellectual. Shepard is action and Hawke is talk. With Shepard as Hawke's father, the complexity and pain in the father/son relationship is made clear.[13]

We learn information about an actor's character by what we know about the actor playing the character next to him.

Or her. When Janet McTeer entered the Delacourt Theatre as Petruchio, the bachelor hoping to "wive it wealthily in Padua" even if it means taming a shrew, the audience had to listen with different interpretive protocols. In Phyllida Lloyd's all-female productions of Shakespeare, the characters remain the same gender even if the actors are clearly a different sex. Both *Julius Caesar* (2014) and *Henry IV* (2014), which started at Donmar Warehouse in London and then moved to St. Ann's Warehouse in Brooklyn, were set in prison. As Michael Billington said in his review of *Julius Caesar*: "the result is a bit like Peter Weiss's *Marat/Sade* in that we are constantly aware of how the drama is shaped by the institutional setting."[14] The casting choice in these two plays partially reflects the limitations of male actors in a women's prison. But the richness of the choice unfolded as the performances went on. As Ben Brantley raved: "It's a multilayered act of liberation. Prisoners are allowed to roam the wide fields of Shakespeare's imagination; fine actresses are given the chance to play meaty roles that have been denied them; and we get to climb out of the straitjackets of our traditional perceptions of a venerated play."[15] Lloyd's productions of *Henry IV* and *Julius Caesar* brilliantly display the horror of the power struggles and the sadness of the bonds made out of institutional alienation and seem to rewrite Shakespeare's "history."

In *The Taming of the Shrew*, however, the "institutional setting" is almost exclusively communicated by the ecology created by the casting. Opening the 2016 season of The Public Theater's Shakespeare in the Park, *Taming of the Shrew* unsettles gender identity, and the politics around it, through casting. Lloyd insisted that she was not willing to soften the misogyny or sadomasochism in the play. At the same time, "Nor will we be wanting to have anything other than quite a riotous night, and I've been lucky enough through The Public to find some extremely funny clowns who will, I hope, help us release cascades of mirth that might not be so easy to access in a more conventionally cast production."[16] This is a strong claim: simply placing female bodies under the male costumes, saying the male lines, helps release "cascades of mirth." Despite a soliloquy/standup routine in which Gremio (Judy Gold) tells sexist jokes while reminding the audience, "You know this show is directed by a woman! They all have boobs!" When one audience member shouted out "Enough with the misogyny!" Gold shouted back: "You feminists have no sense of humor: we're all women, get it?"[17] While the mirth might be a matter of opinion, the nature of Katherine's taming is changed in this ecology of casting.

Katherine's final speech, in which she exhorts women to "place your hands below your husband's foot" (5.2.177), is not easy to recuperate from its misogyny. Delivered by Cush Jumbo as Katherine, who is surrounded by women playing men, the character of the play shifts as character itself seems to be dislocated. Katherine's speech is a long defense of the importance of a gender binary:

> I am asham'd that women are so simple
> To offer war where they should kneel for peace;
> Or seek for rule, supremacy, and sway,
> When they are bound to serve, love, and obey.
> Why are our bodies soft and weak and smooth,
> Unapt to toil and trouble in the world,
> But that our soft conditions and our hearts
> Should well agree with our external parts?
> Come, come, you forward and unable worms!
> My mind hath been as big as one of yours,
> My heart as great, my reason haply more,
> To bandy word for word and frown for frown;
> But now I see our lances are but straws,
> Our strength as weak, our weakness past compare,
> That seeming to be most which we indeed least are.
> (5.2.161–175)

Shakespeare's rhetorical tools (antithesis, rhyme, chiasmus, metaphor, rhetorical question, epanalepsis) are polished and deployed in the service of arguing that biology is destiny in matters of matrimony. As I watched Jumbo/Katherine give this speech on a stage filled with bodies that were all sexed female at birth and that now show a wide variety of shapes and strengths, not to mention costumes, manners, and behaviors, I was unable to find the binary the speech referred to, and as a result, the character itself fell apart. There could be no tamed Kate without a patriarchy-wielding Petruchio. At the end of the speech, Jumbo/Katherine begins screaming and ripping her clothes off and she is caught, held, and placed down the trap as if in a cell. The character of Kate is no more; the ensemble of *Shrew* has made her position untenable. As spectators, we navigate the fictional reality according to what we find in that world, building up strategies and expectations from each choice we encounter. This is one aesthetic consequence of understanding cognition as embodied and embedded. In Lloyd's *Taming of the Shrew*, the all female casting disrupts our protocols of character interpretation because we cannot find the categories of sex and gender the play insists on and thus the *ensemble* stages a character breakdown.

As I watched *Shrew*, I felt the erosion of character because the staging of gender kept challenging what the characters were saying. The bodies of the actors were continually made visible—"they all have boobs!"—and yet there was a wide range of gender performances. On the one hand, this demonstrates the breakdown of gender binaries and the single relationship between bodies sexed male being masculine and bodies sexed female being feminine. On the other hand, because all these female bodies were playing varying genders in a story that is both about and apologizes for patriarchy and misogyny, the category of character is less important here than the story they come together to tell. Most contemporary directors attempt to explain away Kate's taming to mitigate the misogyny: some portray a sadomasochistic pleasure in this couple and others suggest that Kate is faking it, winking at the audience, during that last speech and only playing the game. Lloyd refuses both of those options and by doing so calls the spectator's attention to the belief that Kate and Petruchio cannot be assessed apart from their environment.

Speaking Parts

Eve Ensler's *The Vagina Monologues* started as a one-woman show in New York City in 1996. Ensler performed monologues that she wrote based on interviews with many different women; over the course of the evening, she played women of different ages and backgrounds while sitting barefoot on a stool in a black leotard and skirt. Framing the performance as the result of interviews, Ensler casts herself as the originals, the real people from whom these words have come, instead of casting individual actors to play each part. The women were giving voice, as it were, to only a part of themselves:

> So I decided to talk to women about their vaginas, to do vagina interviews, which became vagina monologues. I talked with over two hundred women. I talked to older women, young women, married women, single women, lesbians, college professors, actors, corporate professionals, sex workers, African American women, Hispanic women, Asian American women, Native American women, Caucasian women, Jewish women. . . . Some of the monologues are close to verbatim interviews, some are composite interviews, and with some I just began with the seed of an interview and had a good time.[18]

These real women are foregrounded before each monologue because feeling the presence of the real women from whom these words, these experiences, have come is key to the impact of the performance. Ensler does not have to convince us that she is these women—in fact, it works almost better when we are aware of the gap between who she is and who the "real" woman was because the gap draws attention to the authenticity of the original. The dispersion of the characters across the same body is part of what generalizes the experience, making the personal political.

In 2000, Ensler stepped down as the performer and replaced herself with three actors, such as Julie Kavner, Swoosie Kurtz, and Audra McDonald, who then would rotate out to make way for another trio of celebrities.[19] According to producer David Stone, "What we have always tried to do when casting these cycles is to have women of different backgrounds and training and constituencies—three women who you might not think would be on a stage together—on a stage together."[20] Ads tempted ticket-buyers with the various celebrities who would "share the microphone at every performance."[21] This was maybe particularly true when Kirstie Alley and Hazelle Goodman were cast with Donna Hanover, wife of New York City mayor Rudy Giuliani. The *New York Times* said: "Call it a bit of political theater or merely some inspired casting, but Donna Hanover's latest acting job might raise some eyebrows at City Hall."[22] Another article in the *New York Times* noted that having his wife talking about vaginas, childbirth, and orgasms onstage each night might create some problems for a Senate run Giuliani was purportedly thinking of.[23] Although Hanover postponed her run in the show when Giuliani announced that he had prostate cancer,[24] she joined a different trio later that year, after her marriage to Giuliani fell apart and Giuliani dropped out of the Senate race. The *New York Times* reporter linked the casting choice to the political environment: "Ms. Hanover's original acceptance of a role in 'The Vagina Monologues' was the first in a chain of events that became part of the mayor's unraveling personal and political life last spring. . . . Few people in political and theatrical circles failed to notice that the play was written by Eve Ensler, a friend and supporter of Hillary Rodham Clinton, who was then Mr. Giuliani's Senate opponent."[25] Casting Hanover to tell the story of a woman gang-raped in Bosnia brought a past political crisis smack into the middle of a current political drama.

Hanover was not herself and also not the Bosnian woman; the casting invited spectators to attend not to individuals but to the mistreated body part they shared. Casting eroded the relationship between a particular woman and a particular story and foregrounded the vacant positions from which any celebrity could speak. They belonged there, speaking those words, because they had a vagina. The simple fact of this physical requirement also foregrounded how this body part united all of the voices in the performance.

Sometimes a detachment between the physical type of the actor and the character—when the actor is clearly not meant to share racial or sexual identifiers with the character—can be productive. This kind of counter casting invites the audience to attend to what matters to them when they build characters. In her documentary, or "verbatim," theater pieces (such as *Fires in the Mirror, Twilight*, and *Lay Me Down*), Anna Deavere Smith plays all the "characters" (the "subjects" of her interviews) with few costumes and in bare feet. She does not become these people—we never forget that it is her up there and not the Rev. Al Sharpton or Texas governor Ann Richards, for example—but she reproduces them, their vocal tics and pauses, in a kind of embodied echo. Smith's acting method repeats, precisely, the sounds and movements of her subject. She does not "become" them psychologically, she incorporates them physically. By foregrounding her own body marked by gender and race while surrendering it to the sounds and tics of her subject, she is staging the interaction *on* and *with* her own body. In that singular body, the audience sees the interviewer, the interviewee, and the audience: it is not a one-woman show; it's a network of organisms, vibrantly coming to life onstage.

Smith has said: "My grandfather told me that if you say a word often enough, it becomes you." And so she is finding her way from her Self to the Other through the words of the others. She goes on to say: "I can learn to know who somebody is, not from what they tell me, but from how they tell me."[26] This is not the reading of text in method acting that analyzes lines for subtext, for what the character feels but is not saying.[27] As Charles Lyons and James Lyons note, "Both Freudian psychology and method acting interpret the surface of speech and gesture as material to be interpreted, to be analyzed and translated. The literal speech and action of a character become secondary, important only as points of access to the real substance of the figure."[28] Method acting thus reflects an older model of how the brain works. It sees it as a kind of algorithmic processing center—the actor enters the given circumstances of the play and her character, sends it through the psychological state of unconscious drives and fears, and then generates behavior. When we watch a film that subscribes to traditional psychological realism, then, this idea is reinforced: we are watching to see an internal function—what caused that stutter? Why is he so mad at women?—an idea of an unconscious inside rather than a cognitive network.

Smith insists that her work is "not psychological realism."

I don't want to own the character and endow the character with my own experience. It's the opposite of that. What has to exist in order to try to allow the other to be is separation between the actor's self and the other. What I'm ultimately interested in is the struggle. The struggle that the speaker has when he or she speaks to me, the struggle that he or she has to sift through language to come through.[29]

We might say that Smith engages in deep surface reading in which she presents the richness of *how* things are said as containing all the information necessary to build a character. Smith honors the salience of "superficial" utterances by attending to the music of the stutters and expressive tics. Her line memorization has been called "a mental martial art;"[30] she repeats the line from the recording of the interview with actors she hires to drill her until the utterance matches—not word for word but "um" for "um." She works to duplicate the "organic poetry" she has heard, not read. She has said: "I think if I'm working well, what people really admire is the effort I'm making to try to leave myself and be someone else."[31] This is, I think, what makes her work funny, what makes it an example of what Gregory Jay calls performative empathy: "Performative empathy is an 'acting out' that includes the cognitive dimension inherent to all emotions, but it is also a 'working through' that challenges us to understand the 'other' through a radical crossing of identity boundaries. Performative empathy helps us see the gap between our own understanding and the perceptions of the subject whom we reenact."[32] What I notice about her casting is her Sisyphean effort to present this politically important black man giving his tribute to James Brown and the ways in which her failure to actually be Rev. Sharpton adds to the beauty of her labor.

She has called acting "the *travel* of the self to the other"— not a becoming of the other or a channeling of the other but a movement between the two.[33] Her language is instructive here because taking her seriously requires a reconceiving of self and other. When I think of myself, I think of the being I do all my traveling in, not something I can travel from. But Smith uses language and acting to imagine and theatricalize just that kind of travel from the self. In discussing her approach to the character of Leonard Jeffries in *Fires in the Mirror*, she told Carol Martin:

> The point is simply to repeat it until I begin to feel it and what I begin to feel is his song and that helps me remember more about his body. For example, I remembered he sat up but it wasn't until well into rehearsal that my body began to remember, not me, my body began to remember. He had a way of lifting his soft palate or something. I can't see it because it's happening inside. But the way it played itself out in early performances is that I would yawn, you know, 'cause he yawned at a sort of inappropriate moment [yawns]. I've realized now what is going on. My body begins to do the things that he probably must do inside while he's speaking. I begin to feel that I'm becoming more like him.[34]

Smith divests herself from her body here, suggesting that there is a body that can remember separate from her. But in this link between her body and his—the sitting up, the lifting of his soft palate—is the portrayal of character. An actor interested in duplicating a kind of internal psychology might read the yawn, the sitting up, for what it *indicated*, as a symptom of internal, subtextual information. Smith simply duplicates the yawn and finds the palate. There is no judgment or narrative, just a struggle to travel from one body to the other, leaving behind her "self"— and staging an alternative to self—in the process. Most articles on Smith or her work talk about its postmodernity, the way the bricolage of voices, the performativity of self, speak to the the-

oretical concerns of the 1990s. Documentary theater challenges
a presumption of a historical truth, and Smith's performances
across race and gender lines do illuminate how the characters are
"playing" their parts for Smith, the interviewer who is playing
her part for them. But Smith stages a shifting epistemology, not
just of history but of self, a self that is dis-individuated from the
body and environment.

Smith's performed interviews generally include a reference
to Smith the interviewer, whose racial/ideological identity the
interviewees are often trying to assess. It is not clear to them
whether she is black, white, or Jewish, and she includes these
confusions in the text of her plays. In *Fires in the Mirror*, Anon-
ymous Black Girl #1 asks, "You black?" Sharpton excludes her
from the white people who have misconceptions about his hair
and a Lubavitcher woman hints that perhaps Smith knows the
rules of the Sabbath. In performance, though, she also needs the
spectator/scholar who, hailed by her text as "you," takes on the
role of the interviewer. Each spectator is then cast as the racially
ambiguous Smith; she must travel between her own self and another. In this performance, spectators can see/feel/hear/know/
experience the radical paradigm and the game-changing possibilities of a redefining and relocating of cognition because they
are in this travel with her. The influence of documentary theater at the end of the twentieth century demonstrates the split
gaze—simultaneously looking at the actor, the character, and
the environment—and the casting unites and stages the three.

The character and the story are not located in an Aristotelian
plot; they are dispersed across networks—the network that connects ideas about hair, say, to the events of Crown Heights. The
literary event is the telling of the story; and it requires Anna Deavere Smith's racial identity just as it requires her bare feet. The
"characters" are not temporarily housed in the body of an actor.
The character of Rev. Al Sharpton or Ann Richards or Mrs. Soon
Young Han is made up of what audience members may know
about the person, the history of the events relevant to the dis-

cussion with Smith, the body of Smith, the virtuosity of Smith's travel, and the relevance of this voice in the story and the moment of performance.

Dispersion

In many contemporary theatrical performances—including *The Vagina Monologues* and the work of Anna Deavere Smith—character is not strictly a combination of the actor and the words written by the playwright. As I argued in chapter 1, the slash between actor and character that I used—Hawke/Hamlet, for example—following Bruce McConachie, to denote this actor's particular version of this character simplifies both character and the work of performance. The enjoyment spectators experience in watching a performance of Deavere Smith is a clear indication that theories of character and casting need to be complicated. An audience member watching Donna Hanover playing a composite Bosnian rape survivor does not build a character so much as perceive the story through more than one storyteller. Characters can be dispersed in performance, and each spectator builds the character from a variety of inputs that come together only in his or her mind. Opera scholar David Levin describes what he calls "dispersion" in the ingredients of character in Pina Bausch's production of C. W. Gluck's *Orpheus and Eurydice*. The "character" was danced by one person and sung by another, thus existing within the spectator as a kind of consolidating entity.[35] This is a useful way to make sense of other contemporary theatrical performances that refuse the binary relationship between actor and character.

Punchdrunk's fantastically successful, immersive performance, *Sleep No More*, opened in an abandoned warehouse in New York City in 2001. Audience members are given masks, taken on an elevator ride, and then let loose to explore three floors of theatrical space. Actors, who are immediately identifiable because they are not wearing masks, dance, interact, speak rarely, and draw individual spectators into private rooms for "one on ones," where the selected spectator might be treated to a story taken from Buchner's *Woyzeck*[36] or pulled nose to nose as the actor whispers "blood will have blood."[37] D. J. Hopkins described it as "a dance theatre adaptation of Shakespeare's *Macbeth*," but the experience feels more Hitchcockian than Shakespearean. W. B. Worthen described the powerful role of the space and the objects as he noted how the performance "reifies Macbeth's interior world as 'immersive' performance space, materializing elements of the play's verbal texture as objects in a thematically resonant environment."[38] Though there are scenes staged between the characters of the play, it is not always easy to keep track of who is playing whom. Because each audience member's experience is different, it is possible to spend an hour wandering the exquisitely designed rooms without finding any evidence of Shakespeare's play. I spent quite some time in a bar watching actors play cards and get into a fight, trying to connect some part of what I was experiencing to *Macbeth*. As Hopkins put it, "Where is Macbeth? I wondered. Where is *Macbeth*, for that matter? *Macbeth* is everywhere and nowhere in *Sleep No More*."[39] Hilton Als credits the relative lack of language for the cohesion of the piece, "Because language is abandoned outside the lounge, we're forced to imagine it, or to make narrative cohesion of events that are unfolding right before our eyes—or on the floor below, without us. We cannot connect with the characters through the thing that we share: language. We can only watch as the performers reduce theatre to its rudiments: bodies moving in space."[40]

Worthen explores the production of character in *Sleep No More*, arguing that it "both charts the pervasive power of long-standing, largely 'literary' conceptions of theatricality to the making of 'new' performance, and—in its dynamic foregrounding of text, character, space, and audience—opens a series of questions about the apparent emancipation of the spectator, and about the character of cognition, offered by theatrical immersion."[41] Worthen uses this production to challenge both criticism of character that "asserts a *realist* understanding of stage performance" and theories of cognitive linguistics applied to theater and performance. In *Sleep No More*, for example, it is not possible to pull Macbeth out of *Macbeth* or to wonder about the Macbeths' lost children. Character here does not line up neatly with Shakespeare's literary text:

> The actors are fully absorbed, meticulously *doing* what they *do*, and even in the scenes more overtly recalling *Macbeth*, much of what they do is not representational, it does not seem to refer to or constitute a fictive person or fictive elsewhere, a *Macbeth, Vertigo, Rebecca*. This concentrated work is astonishing and is perhaps difficult to characterize precisely, because it is not about character; "what the *actor* is *doing*" is what we attend to.[42]

Worthen's insight is critical: despite conventional protocols of narrative meaning-making, *Sleep No More* invites its audience to attend to actions done by actors in a performative environment—actions that are not meant to depict character but are instead meant to build a larger whole, tell a bigger story. I see this as an important way that contemporary performance is asking spectators to reimagine how and through what mechanisms characters can be built. However, where Worthen sees this as a challenge to what he calls the "straightforward blending of literary character to performer described by Fauconnier and Turner," I see it as an opportunity to engage with the cognitive sciences.[43] What does it mean to build characters from the ecosystem up, rather than a more psychologically focused method of character assessment? If thinking is embodied and situated in a particular environment, how might I shift what I can think by shifting what I consider the "location" of a character? The frustrated search for Macbeth in *Sleep No More* suggests that characters may only be one-way spectators who use the environment to think. Theater and performance scholars must extend and complicate what cognitive scientists started, not dismiss such science because it fails to address a particular theatrical experience.

Although those in the arts and humanities have sometimes used blending theory too simplistically, it is not straightforward. As I discussed in the introduction, conceptual integration (blending) theory is a way of explaining how we think in terms of associations, connections, and emergent structure. Blending theory is not about the less complex ideas of "juxtaposition" or "combination." It is a theory of how we think and speak about things, whether those thoughts and words be banal, poetic, or novel. Researchers in the cognitive sciences do not publish on this topic to explain theater or character but rather to use empirical research in neuroscience and linguistics to make sense of the things we say and understand. But blending is a cognitive act we perform each time we see a performance. When Lady Macbeth calls on the spirits to "unsex" her, actors and spectators understand that she is asking for the kind of gender transformation she thinks is required to perform the regicide she is plotting. When we (or Fauconnier and Turner) talk about characters, we are trying to understand not Odysseus and fiction or theater but rather how we can conceptualize a semi-stable entity across time, space, and media. For example, we can read a sentence like "For we have closely sent for Hamlet hither, / That he, as 'twere by accident, may here / Affront Ophelia" (3.1.29–31) and know that "he"— even though it is a different word and in a different part of the sentence—is the same person referred to earlier as "Hamlet." The same thing that guides the child to understand how pronouns work grammatically is the same process that allows the spectator to know that the "he" that enters the stage in act one is the same one that enters in act two.

What cognitive mechanism holds ideas about character together? Why should we think that the words on the page assigned to "Odysseus" or "Hamlet" should have anything to do with the guy we met a minute ago? Humans have an ability to develop a "mental space" called "Hamlet" or "Odysseus" that can be primed or brought to bear at any moment and that carries associations about what that "character" means.

Like characters in *Sleep No More*, Michelangelo's Mary also disrupts what Worthen sees as the "straightforward blending of literary character to performer."[44] Nicolas Moschovakis argues that the clown character in *Titus Andronicus* would have been understood in its original performance in part because of the actor playing the part (Will Kempe) and in part because the play alludes to the hanging of William Hacket for treason.[45] In other words, spectators would have built a rich character that exceeded the matching between character and performer even without a staging that shifted attention from character to environment. Integration networks are a central feature of the cognitive apparatus of homo sapiens; they provide us with a flexible and creative mechanism of compression and connection to make sense of dispersed character information. What is useful to me about conceptual integration theory is the way it provides a rubric for understanding the ways these different input spaces operate to compose meaning.

To understand the composition of meaning is to see it as something we can compose differently. To see Mary or Macbeth as an integration network prompted by the artist(s) is to see other ways the character might have been built. If characters are built, then they can be rebuilt; we need not be passive receivers of characters. The performances I have analyzed in this chapter are vehicles for cognitive change: they push us to see the construction of our integration networks and help us to imagine new cognitive spaces. How might we continue, as theater scholars and practitioners, to use the dispersion of characters and casting that attends the audience to the construction of character to push back against norms of race, gender, and identity?

Contemporary theatrical productions that seem to disperse character across different actors or modalities challenge our seemingly confident assumption that we understand what "character" is to begin with. The masks the spectators are required to wear in *Sleep No More* differentiate the performers from the characters. For Hopkins, the masks are critical to its success: "It depends not only on obsessively dense scenic design, admirable choreography, and an inventive appropriation of a classic text, but on serious thought given to the role of the audience; it turned us into active voyeurs rather than passive consumers."[46] Hilton Als suggests that "to see the various characters without masks—or wearing their characters' face—makes our masked faces look and feel more theatrical and fake than the performers'."[47] Those who are not wearing masks are characters and those of us who are wearing masks are not. This reversal of the conventional use of masks challenges our sense of what's authentic, who is hiding something, and where the characters are. Walking among the spectators, I cannot distinguish between us; we are dis-individuated. I may be able to connect the non-mask wearers to their characters (admittedly, I had a harder time doing this than most of the reviewers or people to whom I spoke), but this is less central to the performance than the erasure of my character as I explore this Macbeth World. By the end of my time in the McKittrick Hotel, I wondered if the idea of stable characters— this one discreet from that one—was the concept to jettison.

CHAPTER 4

CASTING AND THE
PERFORMANCE OF EVERYDAY LIFE

I have argued that casting is a form of dimensionality reduction: all that the actor is and has been and all that the character could be gets reduced when *this* actor takes *this* role at *this* time. I have argued that casting is always ecological: the historical, social, cultural, and political contexts of the choice will always have an impact on the story this actor tells as this character in this moment. Focusing attention on casting exposes the various ways we make characters out of the people around us. While some characters come from fiction and others come from nonfiction, the process of building them remains the same. When I choose my costume in the morning, I am hoping to facilitate my casting as a professor and authority figure. "Dress for the job you want" is good advice because an interview is a casting session. Of course, no outfit can change the way my race helps me or my gender hurts me. Most of the time, this kind of discussion ends in a recognition of racism, sexism, ageism, or, at the very least, implicit bias. These are critically important ideas in contemporary society, but thinking theatrically gives me room to perform differently. When I perform my role as professor, for example, I might reference my love of rap music or the fact that I'm also a mother. I call attention to my white skin while giving a lecture about black theater history. I want students to challenge the character they are building for me and to question the usual "casting" of professors, intellectuals, or older white ladies.

Over the last sixty years, there have been many theoretical and practical demonstrations of the performance of self. One example is the performance of the role of scientist. Stephen Hilgartner has argued that the performance of scientific expertise is a carefully constructed dramaturgy of authority, secrecy, and personae: "These performers [scientists] do not simply appear before audiences; they construct the personae they display, managing information and appearances in complex ways."[1] The influential implication in Hilgartner's work, which is supported by research in psychology, cognitive science, and theater studies, is that information is always processed in relation to our perception of the performer. Spectators do not take in information independent of context, speaker, background, facial expressions, physical gestures, and prosody. This should not be dismissed as superficial or as the influence of bias. Of course, it isn't necessarily true that how we process these factors *isn't* evidence of bias, but we should take them seriously because combating bias requires us to engage with them with a critical eye. Making sense of how we make these judgments about other people—and ourselves—can suggest ways of making smarter judgments.

Understanding the performance of everyday life through the lens of casting gives me tools for thinking my way out of certain casting mistakes. When I speak of casting here, I am not referring to work done by a casting director but rather the "casting" I do when I see that man in a white coat and assign him the role of doctor, authority figure, scientist. A strategic attention to performances—in fiction or in life—that don't seem right, that stretch, extend, or break what seems like the right casting, allows us to see casting as a way to blur or transform categories. People who play against a role, inviting an audience to build a new character through a different performance, can force spectators to consciously think about the role instead of reflexively relying on preexisting cognitive maps. Alternatively, a person who finds herself "cast" by circumstance to play a particular role in a particular narrative may find that the experience alters her self-narrative and transforms her. Casting is creative and ideological, and understanding how it shapes our everyday life grants us an indirect way of thinking about our thinking and the opportunity—perhaps our responsibility—to change what we think.

Casting Is Candidate Selection

Americans would like to believe that they choose a candidate for president based on who makes the best arguments or advances the best policies. Candidate selection can be viewed as a type of casting: politicians attempt to show that they can play the role and voters look for information about a candidate that makes him or her ineligible to play the part of president. Citizens build characters that fit the role of president and view the ones they do not like as not fitting that role. Voters seek a leading man or woman to play a theatrical role: Which actor who is auditioning "feels right" as the next head of state? The winning candidate best fits the way voters wish to imagine the "movie" of the next four years of their lives. In 2005, researchers found that "rapid automatic inferences from the facial appearance of political candidates can influence processing of subsequent information about these candidates."[2] This data led the researchers to predict fairly accurately which candidate would win a hypothetical election. Later fMRI studies have suggested that the bilateral amygdala is more active in response to faces of the politicians subjects planned to vote for, independent of the subject's—or the candidate's—culture.[3] Psychologist Drew Weston and colleagues reported that while participants in an fMRI study watched video of potentially damaging political information about the political candidates they preferred, the part of the brain associated with reasoning was calm and the parts associated with emotions were active.[4] This, he concludes, is evidence that emotions play a central role in candidate selection. It also suggests that once voters have selected someone they feel is right for the part, they are hesitant to challenge this match.

Once we have categorized a person as favorable, electable, right to be president, we come to see this view as objective. This actor is an ingénue, this actor is a clown, and this politician is presidential. Our category of "president" is not based on a set of conditions that must be met if we are to include a candidate in that category (intelligence, experience, policy insight, leadership); it is based on that candidate's similarity to the prototypes we have constructed. The prototypical U.S. president may look like Michael Douglas or Ronald Reagan, but that doesn't mean that someone like Franklin D. Roosevelt or Barack Obama might not fit. Categories do not expand easily, however, because people assume they are based on an objectively assessed set of shared properties. If that is the case, then changing what or who belongs in the category is not easily done. On the other hand, seeing candidates as performers might make it easier for voters to expand what or who belongs in their category.

In much the same way that spectators build fictional characters based on the previous roles an actor has played that are ghosting his current performance, political candidates refer to past performances as evidence of their suitability. During the 2016 election, Hillary Clinton often reminded voters of her performance in the Situation Room as key members of the Obama administration waited to hear the results of the raid on the Osama bin Laden compound. Many of Donald Trump's previous performances—on *The Apprentice*, with the Miss Universe contest, and so forth—struck many voters as evidence of his unsuitability for presidency, but it turns out that these previous roles made Trump seem powerful, decisive, and attractive to a section of American voters. Some baggage, even scandals or addictions, can be good press because it makes for good drama. While the scope of what we can forgive evolves with time, Americans have always loved redemptions. Some of our favorite actors have been warmly received when they came back from personal debacles. Robert Downey Jr.'s history of arrests and drug addiction (and recovery) made him the superpower that could turn *Iron Man* into the highest grossing film of 2013 ($1.2 billion). Hugh Grant's public arrest on Sunset Strip only added to his awkward charm in *Notting Hill* (1999). And audiences love movies about coming back from a low point. According to a 2004 BBC poll, *It's A Wonderful Life* (1946) was voted the second-best movie never to win an Oscar; *The Shawshank Redemption* (1994) was rated the highest in this category. Just as we build the characters of our fictional heroes, we build the character of the political candidates we consider, and complexity, drama, and layers can be compelling.

The fact is the most trusted man in America is not Bernie Sanders or Donald Trump. It is Tom Hanks. The Marketing Arm is a company that claims to "harness the power of emotion to make brands more engaging," partially through assessing the perceived credibility of different celebrities clients might think to sell their products."[5] Talking to Scott Simon of NPR, Matt Delzell of The Marketing Arm said, "It's saddening to know that the top ten in trustworthiness includes mostly actors. And we're talking about, you know, again, people who play fictitious characters that other people write for them."[6] The characters that Hanks plays have so infused our creation of his actual character that we fail to distinguish between the two.

Casting and Category Confusion

It is reasonable to assume that a sizable portion of the voting public was never able (or willing) to see Barack Obama as president. They perceived him as being fundamentally miscast because, for them, being a white male feels like one of the necessary and sufficient conditions of a U.S. head of state. The first time Barack Obama performed the role of the president who gives the State of the Union address in 2009, Representative Joe Wilson miscast the president of the United States as a man standing on a soapbox, inviting dialogue and debate rather than respectful attention. For Wilson, President Obama's casting so confused his category of president that he failed to perform the basics of decorum and respect. Many Americans believed that the casting

of Barack Obama as president profoundly changed the conceptual category of president. For them, because Obama successful-
ly ran for and played the part, the role was changed. For other
voters, Obama could never be "their president" because they see
categories as fixed and have less experience with category expansion. During the 2016 election, they felt the need to "take their
country back" and "make it great again" because the miscasting
of president was a sure sign that it had been taken and was no
longer great. Although some of this is racism—and sexism—it is
also category confusion.[7] When the issue is understood this way,
it might be easier to confront and address.

One way to address category confusion is through storytelling and rehearsal. Casting directors give us pivotal information
about the story we are being told by whom they select to play the
parts. Lori McCreary, Morgan Freeman's producing partner in
Revelations Entertainment and president of the Producers Guild
of America, told the *New York Times*: "If [a script doesn't specify,
a role is] presumed to be white and male. For *Deep Impact*, Mimi
Leder, the director, wanted to cast Morgan as the president, and
somebody at the studio said, we're not making a science-fiction
movie; you can't have Morgan Freeman play the president. But
she really fought for it."[8] When black actor Dennis Haysbert was
cast as presidential candidate David Palmer in the TV program
24, spectators understood that the series was set in the near future. As Brandi Wilkins Catanese argues, "Consumption of images of black presidents offers American audiences the opportunity
to rehearse acceptance of a black person in perhaps the most im-
probable role available in America (or to confirm such a turn of
events as a dystopic national condition)."[9]

The American electorate had consumed many images of female presidents and female authority figures, and for many, it
confirmed a "dystopic national condition" that was similar to
how they received the Obama presidency. I, and many others,
found ourselves surprised by our own confirmation bias; for us,
Hillary Clinton's performance during the Benghazi hearings and
in debates against Donald Trump produced what casting direc-

tors would call a reel: hours and hours of the actor/candidate demonstrating her ability to play the part that she is up for. Her performance of the role gave spectators an opportunity to, as Catanese puts it, "rehearse acceptance" of women as heads of state. Casting directors know that you can, with care, bring an audience to expand their categories. When Judi Dench became Bond's M in 1995, spectators recognized her authority, intelligence, and experience as close enough to the prototypical M that her gender was uncontroversial. Although the casting of Dench may have been uncontroversial—as opposed to, say, the all-female remake of *Ghostbusters* (2016)—it does not mean that other characters in Bond films didn't "mansplain" to Dench/M about espionage or interrupt her in meetings, or that Dench the actor was paid the same as her male counterparts.

The problem is, according to Virginia Valian, that both men and women have gender schemas—"intuitive hypotheses about the behaviors, traits, and preferences of men and women, boys and girls"—that "affect our expectations of men and women, our evaluations of their work, and their performance as professionals."[10] These are almost like the "casting breakdowns" that give casting directors shorthand descriptions of parts ("In his 40s, a rumpled and sleepless Communications Director at the White House"). These schemas make it very difficult to perceive women as competent when they perform in roles we do not expect them to excel in. Valian tracks how this shapes gender enculturation at school, perceptions of women in professions, and the accumulation of disadvantage over time. Her summary of what happens to women in leadership roles won't come as a surprise to many women:

> When women attempt to be leaders they lose, relative to men, in three steps. First, they are attended to less; they have more difficulty than men do in gaining and keeping the floor. Second, when women do speak and behave like leaders, they receive negative reactions from their cohorts, even when the content and manner of their presentations are identical to men's. . . . Third, even observers

with no overt bias are affected by negative reactions to women leaders and tend to go along with the group judgment.[11]

Critically, Valian frames this not as an issue of sexism but rather as an issue of overly generalized and lazy gender schemas. These are schemas we can change and expand with attention, diligence, and creative casting.

Schemas—like categories—are not the problem. They "are a cognitive necessity for making sense of the social world of every day life. Schemas may contain errors, but they are indispensable."[12] One of Valian's "remedies" suggests that we challenge the hypotheses or schemas of ourselves and of those around us. A second suggestion is that we make sure we spend time in places where women are well-represented, since the fewer women, the greater share of bias (to paraphrase Shakespeare's Henry V).[13] Another useful suggestion came from the women of the Obama White House: "When a woman made a key point, other women would repeat it, giving credit to its author. This forced the men in the room to recognize the contribution—and denied them the chance to claim the idea as their own."[14] They called it "amplification." Strategic performances can challenge and extend our schemas and increase the number of roles we think women are capable of playing.

Hillary Clinton acknowledged the power and prevalence of implicit bias in the presidential debate on September 25, 2016: "I think implicit bias is a problem for everyone, not just police. I think unfortunately too many of us in our great country jump to conclusions about each other and therefore I think we need all of us to be asked the hard questions 'why am I feeling this way?'"[15] The next morning The Washington Times ran a headline that read: "Hillary Clinton Calls the Entire Nation Racist."[16] Implicit bias is not racism—which is not to say that it isn't a part of institutional racism. Clinton was giving America the power and the responsibility to examine our biases and our performances, to examine how quickly we may judge another and to push against that. Rick Perry and the man across the street in a hoodie may both be "straight out of central casting" for particular roles, but that does not mean they would be well cast in those roles.

Wearing a hoodie and carrying a bag of Skittles, Trayvon Martin was killed on February 26, 2012, by George Zimmerman. For some, Martin's costume and props became symbols of racial profiling and injustice. Geraldo Rivera said parents should not let their kids wear hoodies, claiming: "I think the hoodie is as much responsible for Trayvon Martin's death as George Zimmerman was."[17] There was a "Million Hoodie March" in New York City and other protests and rallies of support around the country. In March, President Obama said, "If I had a son, he'd look like Trayvon. . . . We're going to get to the bottom of exactly what happened."[18] It was at this point, Ta-Nehisi Coates argues, that conservatives began mounting a defense of George Zimmerman and vilifying Martin. Coates argues that President Obama made visible two mental spaces that many Americans never want to see compressed into one character: federal power and black skin:

> The irony of Barack Obama is this: he has become the most success-
> ful black politician in American history by avoiding the radioactive
> racial issues of yesteryear, by being "clean" (as Joe Biden once la-
> beled him)—and yet his indelible blackness irradiates everything
> he touches. . . . But when President Barack Obama pledged to "get
> to the bottom of exactly what happened," he was not protesting or
> agitating. He was not appealing to federal power—he was employ-
> ing it. . . . Barack Obama governs a nation enlightened enough to
> send an African American to the White House, but not enlightened
> enough to accept a black man as its president.[19]

Obama generally did not "stage" or foreground his race in rela-
tion to his position of power the way he did in this moment. In this moment, what some in America viewed as a "miscasting" (a black man as president) was salient in a new way in the national dialogue. What became visible was that many Americans see

"white" as an essential characteristic of a president. Categories are based on prototypes, and what feels like "miscasting" to one group might eventually cause the category to expand and change.

While racial profiling, which quickly casts certain people as having a particular story, is an example of cognitive efficiency—overgeneralizing data to save time, that does not mean it is accurate or the right way to move forward. These reactions are often automatic and unconscious; one study revealed that both white and black officers shot faster at images of people with dark skin than those with light skin.[20] The efficiency categorization and schemas provides must be offset by an effort to reperform and recast our roles. Racial profiling leads to more than just an accumulation of disadvantage. In the "hey you" with which the police hail the young black man walking home at night, the police cast him as a threat because of the color of his skin. This inability of the police officer to challenge and extend his conceptual categories of threat and criminal can have serious consequences.

Casting Is Transformative

Language and performance create a narrative that produces entailments; what logically follows from the "casting" of Trayvon as a criminal by Zimmerman or the "casting" of Trayvon as the son of Obama may be different but both are powerful. Language and performance also obscures connections and shapes assumptions about characters. The story Obama told about seeing Trayvon Martin as someone who could have been his son changed the character that some people had created for their president. Suddenly, in their minds, he was the angry and wronged father of a black man who had the power of the United States military behind him. Obama changed the narrative, and narratives change characters. Patrick Colm Hogan argues that "every structure are fundamentally shaped and oriented by our emotion systems" and that stories may even be a "necessary part of the development of our emotional lives."[21] Stories make us feel, and the emotions they invoke shape how we see the characters involved in the stories. Hogan's insight into the relationship between emotions, stories, and characters is informative. He argues that stories can inform how we respond to others:

> There are ways in which our emotional responses—including our empathetic responses—may be attenuated or enhanced. In part, such modulations result from interpretive processes—just the sort of processes we cultivate in literary study. In this way, our emotional responses to stories—thus our emotional memories—are not only a matter of what is in the stories but also how we think about what is in the stories."[22]

A story can cast characters and evoke emotions.

During a debate about a bill that sought to restrict access to abortions on the floor of the Michigan House in 2012, State Representative Lisa Brown referred to her vagina and all hell broke loose. She was banned from speaking the next day. One Republican lawmaker told the press, "What she said was offensive. It was so offensive, I don't even want to say it in front of women. I would not say that in mixed company."[23] This incident garnered state and national attention for Brown, and Eve Ensler showed up to spend a week performing *The Vagina Monologues* on the House steps. Many were shocked that the word "vagina" on its own could be perceived as so dangerous. I suggest that the furor was not about her specific language. (Although I doubt that the word "penis" would have been welcomed on the floor of the House, the comparison is hard to investigate since penises are rarely the subject of legislation.) Representative Brown cast herself and her colleagues in untenable ways, and her performance was far enough out of role to cause furor.

Representative Brown gave an intelligent and impassioned speech on the proposed law, discussing it in terms of loss of jobs, costs to voters, and religious freedom.[24] She pointed out that although her Jewish faith values the life of the mother over the fetus in these cases, she was not asking them to adhere to her

religious perspective and asked why they were asking her to adhere to their religious views. Then she added, "And finally, Mr.
Speaker, I'm flattered that you're all are so interested in my vagina, but 'no' means 'no.'"[25] There are several ways that viewing
this performance through the lens of casting can help us see the
potential of transformational casting. First, by referring to "my"
vagina, Brown foregrounded her sex on the floor of the House,
casting her as a female colleague, the kind of colleague who—
for some—turns "company" into "mixed" company. Second, the
"no means no" comment evoked a scenario in which she was attempting to stop a rape. This script cast her as the victim and
them as perpetrators; any attempt to continue to lobby for their
bill became a kind of forced penetration after that remark. Third,
her stepping out of her role—transforming from dispassionate
legislator to emotional feminist—forced a category change for
the "mixed company" of the floor, a situation that was met with
opprobrium, if not horror.

The first two points altered the casting through the connection Brown made between rape and abortion legislation. An attempt to legislate abortion is clearly not the same as rape, but
Brown's blend masked the differences while highlighting—and
generating—similarities. In the rape space, penetration of the
vagina is done against the will of the woman for the purposes of
the perpetrator's pleasure. The victim says no in order to clearly
indicate her lack of consent and thus to mark the event as a rape.
In the space of legislated abortion, there is a procedure that relates to the product of intercourse and involves the vagina, but
the penetration involved, which the woman seeking the abortion
is requesting, is being stopped by the lawmakers against the will
of the woman. In the blend, Brown's statement that "no means
no" marked an attempt to legislate abortions as a violating act
similar to rape. Her language forcefully cast her male colleagues
by generating a network that connected their actions as lawmakers to the criminal acts of rapists and her action of speaking on
the floor of the house to the cry of a potential victim.

The attention male legislators paid to Brown's use of the word "vagina" obscured what made the performance so powerful: by casting herself and the situation differently, Brown invited her colleagues to react differently—and they did, by banning her. Even so, by spinning a different tale and taking on a different part, the space was made for other performances, other parts to play. Being banned is the evidence that with her abrupt category changes—from legislator to feminist and from legislator to potential rape victim—Brown succeeded in stepping out of her place.

A story is not the same as an event. In the same way that Obama's hypothetical scenario about Trayvon Martin is not the same as his actually being the father of a murdered son, being raped is different from evoking the narrative for political purposes. Rape is a performance that transforms through casting. The damage it can do to a person is below the perception of our legal system because it is a violence to identity, not just to the body. Once you have been a rape victim, there is no removing that role from your character: you are never *not* the person who had this traumatic experience. Kim Solga talks about the metatheatrical return of rape, particularly in the drama and performance of the early modern period. She points out that "rape creates a fundamental epistemological dilemma" because it is inner and is defined not by the act but by the desires and intentions of those involved.[26] After a rape, nothing is missing, yet everything is different. For Solga, the "world-breaking self-loss that marks the experience of rape" is partially due to the performance required of the woman in order to obtain justice.[27] It is only a rape if she adequately performs her "hue and cry":

> Only after a victim has properly performed her trauma for "the good men of the next towne" can she sue to the authorities; the performance *makes the crime actionable*. Just as in the theatre, where the heroine's "return" to the stage post-rape stands in for an act that exists only as a gap in the story, the carefully scripted telling of rape transforms the crime from an event with little epistemic status (an event *of* the woman's body) into an event *of* public space, and *for* the men who guard that space.[27]

While Solga is specifically speaking of the laws of the early modern period, the performances of trauma that are often required of contemporary women suggest that this remains a part of the story of rape. This is Brown's necessary cry of "no means no," which casts her as an unwilling victim rather than as a willing participant.

In order to make the perpetrator into a villain, the woman must be the victim. She is forcefully involved in a duet of male pleasure and female torture in which rape requires and then rejects her, and she loses agency over her body. She is recast. Forever after, this is now one of the things that can happen to her, one of the roles she has played. Emma Sulkowicz dramatized this at Columbia University. When the administration would not expel the man she identified as her rapist, she began carrying her mattress everywhere she went. She was never not performing the role he cast her as: responsible for and attached to the bed it happened on. The performance garnered her media attention and provoked a countersuit from the young man. Sulkowicz's actions made the entire campus witness to her trauma. She harnessed the power of casting by transforming her response to her experience into a performance that attempted to cast every person on campus as either a villain or a witness.[28] The *New York Times* followed up on this story in July of 2017 with the headline: "Columbia Settles with Student Cast as a Rapist in Mattress Act Project."[30]

We cast others and we have the power to miscast and recast them. Sulkowicz's and Brown's performances pushed back. Brown may have been banned by the men in the room, but many others came to see the clashing narratives and counter-performances as illuminating. Why shouldn't she be also an angry feminist with a vagina on the floor of the House? Some category change may happen with a ban and others may happen slowly, performance after performance after performance. Patterns are made and change over time.

CHAPTER 5

COUNTER CASTING
Building Colony

Meryl Streep gave a workshop for a small group of graduate and undergraduate theater students at Indiana University in 2014. I asked her how she thinks about herself in relationship to the characters she chooses to play, and she said, "every new person I'm going to make is on the caboose of a lot of other people but they are all me."[1] I imagined her crafting characters and attaching them to a growing train of cars—each car another other character she's played before—and becoming a more and more powerful train the more cars she adds. When pressed to elaborate on this train image, she decided the train wasn't the right metaphor but rather that all the characters were in her to begin with. Now I imagined a very big green room, filled with different potential characters for Streep to play. The two different metaphors she used for acting are helpful points of interrogation: Does she, Streep, grow like a train the more characters she portrays, or has she always had a large number of distinct characters within her? Do we all have this potential multitude or is she particularly talented at finding and unearthing these internal characters?

In this final chapter, I challenge the parameters of self and how casting might provide a way of refusing the roles we are given, the stories we are told. Can casting counter our way of thinking? Attending to moments of surprise, discomfort, or confusion in the theater might open up a space where we can be something different, where we can shift our attention away from who we are as individuals and toward the purpose we serve in the group. Theater, like the arts in general, reflects current scientific truths: as Joseph Roach pursued in *The Player's Passion* and R. Darren Gobert argued in *The Mind-Body Stage*, acting stages the scientific understanding of the playwright and actors. By doing so, it can also generate stories and metaphors—ways of seeing—for its spectators. One contemporary performance moved me in such a way as to open up a new way of thinking about where and who I was. We think we are individuals with stable essences, but what if there's another way to cast ourselves? What if something else is equally true?

Staging Science

How we tell stories changes how we see ourselves. R. Darren Gobert argues that theater after Rene Descartes reflected a concept of interiority and the importance of passions: actors were prized for displaying: "In theater after Descartes, actors came to be evaluated not only for their outward abilities to represent emotion but for their interior perceptual, emotional, and volitional apparatuses, which determine these outward abilities and shape their performative expression."[2] Gobert refutes the reading of Descartes as separating the body and the mind popularized by Antonio Damasio's book, *Descartes' Error*. In fact, argues Gobert, Descartes saw the "animal spirits" as uniting the body, mind, and passions. While contemporary scientists might point to a lack of evidence for "animal spirits," Gobert reads Descartes as committed to a mind-body union: "Descartes defines the emotions as bodily perceptions and thus precisely as a source of knowledge. . . . Failing to understand the workings of mind-body union, critics [   ] misread Descartes's concept of mind but also miss the crucial role that the passions play in the process of reason."[3] The cultural shift engendered by Descartes in this area is most vibrantly evident at the theater. He finds in Corneille's "deviation from classical form" a turn to "wonder," "the precise emotion that Descartes located at the center of his emotional physics and moral philosophy"; he explores Racine's *Phedre* as a demonstration of the power of the passions to overcome the body and argues that "perspectival staging seemed to promise the ontological security of the spectator."[4]

In his chapter on Cartesian Acting, Gobert argues that one example of the influence of Descartes on theater is the casting of actors to play themselves. He argues that Moliere's *The Versailles Impromptu* brilliantly confuses actors and characters by naming many of the characters the names of the actors playing them. This "Pirandellian trick" provides a "theoretical means and motivation for the performer" to act as naturally as possible because "the individual actor is licensed to make himself or herself into a character, both in a literal sense (since Du Parc played 'Du Parc,' for instance) and in a philosophical sense (since the self of the actor, his or her own *caractère*, is to anchor that of the role)."[5] Audiences, aware both of the characters and the actors, are invited to see the characters as more natural because the illusion of "play" has been removed. Du Parc must be perfect inside and out for the part of Du Parc. This metatheatricality in casting is also found on the English stage of George Villiers' *The Rehearsal,* which calls for the entrance of George Shirley, as himself. The actor is already known to the spectators, argues Gobert,

> not as a character but as a three-dimensional person, possessing an interiority and embodying the altogether unique history of his particular past performances . . . . Shirley's cameo has the same theatrical effect as the inappropriate giggles of an actor who breaches the theatrical illusion, what the British call corpsing: the character "dies" as a result of the over-whelming effect of the actor's own agency.[6]

Actors playing themselves delighted the spectators by staging an internal and essential self.[7] Like Roach's argument that theories of acting in the Elizabethan period relied on a Galenic conception

of humors, Gobert's argument points to how scientific conceptions of the self drive, and are reflected in, what's on stage.

Laura Otis demonstrates a similar relationship in the literature and science of the nineteenth century. In *Membranes: Metaphors of Invasion in Nineteenth-Century Literature, Science, and
Politics,* Otis explores how practitioners in various disciplines
used the metaphor of a membrane as a way of perceiving and
generating borders. In the nineteenth century, the language of
membranes permeated Western culture. She sees it in the way
politicians and generals think about national boundaries, in
narratives of exclusion, and in artistic representations of the
self. Key to these modes of thought was the idea of the membrane, that which separated the "pure" from the "impure." The
shift from seeing disease as traveling in the "miasma" to seeing
it as being passed through germs meant that individuals had
germs, not areas. Germs could be visualized and were described
as having a force and as invading people.[8] Seeing membranes and
germs in the nineteenth century provided humans with a narrative of the self that required a policed boundary. She finds this
in the literature of the period as well, with characters like Sherlock Holmes's Watson, weakened by the bullet from abroad as
Sherlock investigates and diagnoses crimes and criminals from
abroad that have gotten in. Although the microscope technology
had been around since 1670, it was the literature of the period,
Otis argues, that circulated the metaphor of membranes that allowed the scientists to see differently what was under their microscope. The relationship between fiction and science has fos-
tered many wonderful discoveries, such as the germ theory of
the nineteenth century. As Otis points out, "Cell theory relies
on the ability to perceive borders, for to see a structure under
a microscope means to visualize a membrane that distinguishes
it from its surroundings." Thus, for Otis, germ theory is a part
of the "culturally motivated enclosure movement" of the nineteenth century.[9]

Germ theory was critical medically, but it was also powerful
ideologically. Otis suggests that biology offers correlates that

are other ways to imagine the relationships between individuals and community. For example, she looks at the physiology of how thought occurs in the brain. Thought occurs, she writes, because neurons are able to "form new connections and associations." Neurons are plastic; they are able to change. But this doesn't happen in isolation; neurons draw upon "the cells to which they are connected and the nature of communication between them."[10] Each connection creates the possibility of new thought. From this example, Otis extrapolates ideas about human communication: "In the same manner, people and nations can define themselves in terms of connections and relationships, so that contact enriches rather than threatens identity."[11] While the language of the self as a container is useful, it obscures some ways of thinking. If we are containers, connections between others are the exception, rather than the rule. If we are containers, knowledge is something that I have within, as opposed to demonstrate in action in the environment. If I thought of myself as a murmuration of starlings, on the other hand, I exist in coordinated action, and dissolve into the environment when not. Just as our conception of the brain as something with thoughts, ideas, and memories stored—or "repressed"—as static percepts in our brain is a historically contingent narrative of the brain, so to is our bounded notion of the individual.

Like Otis, Bruce McConachie is interested in the idea of historically contingent boundaries. He argues that the metaphor of containment structured much of the drama and performance of the Cold War period. McConachie labels characters like Brick in *Cat on a Hot Tin Roof* Empty Boys—their outside presentation belies a tortured or contrasting inside.[12] Characters like Willy Loman in *Death of a Salesman* are Fragmented Heroes: men who are "powerful masters of their fate and impotent in the face of nuclearism," caught in a bunkered family located in a contained nation.[13] These characters, who were portrayed by actors trained in method acting to evoke "emotional memory," offered spectators stories of borders under attack. McConachie connects this way of perceiving and performing characters with a geo-political narrative of countries at risk of invasion and a psychoanalytic story of characters with "superior knowledge and intelligence rendered temporarily impotent by physical or psychological problems."[14] Viewed historically, these characters assume—and perpetuate—a conception of the self with boundaries and depth.

Theatrical characters—at least since Ibsen—have also tended to be individuals. In other words, the dramaturgy attends to the singular man or woman and his or her challenges, psychology, triumph, or fall. When Linda insists at Willy Loman's funeral that "attention must be paid," Arthur Miller, through Linda, is arguing that despite the challenges of the family and changes in economic/social structure of society, the work and value of the *individual* man must be respected. From Shirley's true essence staged in his cameo as Shirley in *The Rehearsal* to the death of Willy Loman in Miller's *Salesman*, characters have been important because they were singular. Characters in theater more recently, however, are not as singular, as I argued about *Sleep No More* and Anna Deavere Smith's plays. Spectators may be hungry for a metaphor of the self that alters the bounded container and these new metaphors are often visible in the casting. Casting that counters a strong narrative about the individual opens up a vision of the community, of who we are as connected neurons, rather than enclosed membranes. Theater gives us a way to stage and reimagine categories like the self during moments when they are placed into flux. The psychological realism of Arthur Miller or Tennessee Williams, a dramaturgy of the internal causes that motivate the individual, is giving way to a theater that shifts our perspective from the "insides" of characters (wherein one finds their history or backstory) to the networks that connect us, that make us enact the event together.

War Horse

I felt, saw, and heard many involuntary reactions to the killing as I sat safely in the Lincoln Center Theater in 2011 watching *War*

Horse. Based on a young adult novel about horses during World War I, the stage play used life-sized puppets, made of wire and netting and manipulated by three visible men, to bring the horses to life. Cast as puppets, the horses nonetheless evoke visceral reactions from the audience when they are hurt onstage by the actors/characters with whom they perform. I was not the only one who flinched and squirmed in my seat when the soldier plunged the knife into a horse's head or when horses were caught in barbed wire. My body was never in danger and there was no real horse. The audience knew that a horse had died when the puppeteers extricated themselves from the puppet shell and left the stage. I did not believe that a horse died, and yet that might have been the most powerful staging of death that I've ever experienced.

As my body flinched and clenched, I could see and feel spectators around me respond similarly. In his review, Ralf Remshardt noticed the audience's reaction to the perceived pain "experienced" by inanimate objects on stage: "When the horses were seen to suffer—there was a chilling scene in which they got caught in barbed wire—the audience suffered audibly as well."[15] Most theories of narrative empathy or emotion suggest that we believe that the fictional world is real and therefore feel real emotions about an unreal event.[15] I do not think that a spectator could believe that there were real horses onstage being hurt. I believe that the response is both greater and smaller than the one suggested by Samuel Taylor Coleridge's "willing suspension of disbelief."[17] Coleridge formulates belief as the regular state of being but that we can put it on temporary hold in order to believe what is not true. I resist this formulation in part because it offers little hope for change: what happens in the theater can stay in the theater because all "belief" was suspended. As psychologist Richard Gerrig argues, it is actually disbelief that must be constructed: our default position is to believe what we are told in fiction; Gerrig and David Rapp found that when subjects were transported by a narrative, they were more likely to be persuaded by the conclusions of the story—even when they were told the stories were false.[18] Through effort, we can use our better natures to change what we believe. Empathy, a feeling with someone or something else, can bring us to change our minds with and through our hearts.[19]

This feeling of empathy must explain why people will spend money to have the experience of suffering. Why else would audiences enjoy watching aversive stimuli? From *Oedipus* to *Nightmare on Elm Street* to *War Horse*, people have come together to watch people pretend to be in pain. The squirm of empathetic pain, that flinch when we guard our groin despite the fact that it is only happening on the screen in front of us, returns us to our bodies in our seats. The body adjusts as it squirms, and I feel my muscles tense and the boundaries of my body return to my perception. I can tell that it is not my body that is in danger. I did not squirm because I thought I was actually in danger, I squirmed in empathetic response to the aversive stimuli. What was my response to this experience? Did I tell others that they should not see this play because of the intensity of the experience? No; just the opposite. I told them all that they too had to experience that precious torture. The empathy I was reminded of when I squirmed is part of the work of theater: I could feel for the character onstage and I had make sense of that experience.

But how does the process of making sense of the intense discomfort of the visceral squirm work? In her book on visual art, Jill Bennett argues that the squirm is "a moment of regrouping the self," a sensation that "works with and against" a deeper-level response that is unbearable "on its own." For Bennett, the recoil is "not a retreat but a way of negotiating the felt impact of the image." It gives us time to "locate ourselves in relation to the image" and "inure ourselves to its effects."[20] In other words, the involuntary squirm gives us a chance to become accustomed psychologically to the stimulus that generates such a powerful physical response. The squirm opens up a space where the limits of the self are negotiable—there is pain and I must work to clarify that it's not me, but in that moment I can think about me as bigger, more.

If we can allow new information in through those cracks, it is just possible that we can change how we think about ourselves, and if we can do that, we can change how we think about others. The first step in that process is seeing our connections, our similarities to those we think of as "other." In order to understand my reaction to the knifed horse puppet, I had to question the assumption of individuality. The fact that I felt along with that puppet suggests that my ability to feel pain and experience life is far more expansive than the boundary of my body. My squirm reaction was information that told me that I was undergoing that process of feeling *with* someone or something beyond the boundaries of my own experience, beyond the boundaries of my own body. I was in new territory. This is precisely the way that counter casting, where actors and characters are not where or whom I expect, opens up a space where things can be different. It requires a reevaluation of self and other.

Empathy cracks open our illusion that we are safe, that we are separate. In her essay on empathy and watching differently abled dancers, Wanda Strukus argues that "the experience of watching performers with different physical abilities can contribute to changing our perceptions about physical difference."[21] Her ideas about this physical, mirroring of feeling with and through the movements of others are based in part on mirror neuron research. Strukus calls it "kinesthetic empathy" and cites research that shows that some people—dancers for example—score higher on tests of kinesthetic empathy than others.[22] Nonetheless, kinesthetic empathy can engage and change our minds in part because it has the capacity to engage both nonconscious and conscious processes.

We may not always be aware of the ways in which our perspectives are being reinforced or changed through exposure to movement. The plasticity of the brain allows for change, and the act of merely watching the movement of a differently-abled body may contribute or instigate change, but it seems clear that the movement watched must be authentic to the differently-abled body that performs it.[23]

Wheelchair dancers experience the wheelchair as part of their body and can perceive the difference between how an able-bodied dancer and a disabled-bodied dancer use a wheelchair. For spectators without an extended experience of the body in a wheelchair, the chair used by another may seem like an "object or a piece of equipment that a person is in or on, separate from the body itself and symbolic of disability."[24]

This misunderstanding, Strukus thinks, is part of what allowed the creators of *Glee* to cast a non-disabled actor to play the part of Artie, a disabled teen. For the disabled community, Artie's performance "felt" wrong; he did not seem to dance in his chair like someone for whom the chair is an extension of self. Strukus quotes one blogger: "There's absolutely no body-chair integration at all. They [non-disabled performers] think of sitting in a chair as being only about not being able to move their legs."[25] This casting choice was a missed opportunity to expose viewers' to the subtle, perhaps imperceptible to some, differences in how differently abled bodies use a wheelchair when they dance. The casting of an able-bodied actor in this role allowed spectators to continue to believe that they know what the experience is, that it was accessible to them with an imagination and a chair. But it is precisely the gap between where I am and where my empathy goes—to a body that feels different or three men operating a puppet—that encourages new connections and requires that I rethink my assumptions in order to make sense of this novel experience. Strukus calls this "mining the gap" between our own experience and those of others. This comes about, I suggest, through strategic casting.

As I sat in the audience for *War Horse*, feeling with the horse, surrounded by other audience members who were similarly "audibly suffering" with the horse, I tried to understand what cognitive work might be being done in the system we were in, the space of the theater in that moment. What was it about that play that caused us to feel such a visceral sense of empathy? On my way to and from Lincoln Center, I witnessed (although I ignored) many instances of suffering that I did not experience as profoundly as

I experienced the death of a puppet on stage, so clearly it is not the fact of suffering alone that pulls us in. Those who saw it with me that night said that we felt with the horse because it was so lifelike. That was reviewer Remshardt's experience as well: "As in Bunraku, once the illusion is established, they appear as real as if they were the animal itself."[26] I disagree. It was not that I believed that the horse was alive; it was that I knew the horse was not alive and squirmed when it suffered anyway. I felt empathy for what was onstage regardless of what it was, and that, to me, is far more moving than the idea that a powerful illusion was created. The illusion theory, the "suspension of disbelief" theory, suggests that had they stabbed a real horse, I would have felt even more. That action would have required vastly different actions: uproar, storming the stage, etc. Counter casting, in this case casting three men in a wire cage to play a horse, was what brought meaning to my squirm.

When the men withdrew from the horse-cage, signifying the horse's death, I saw a network of forces engaged in bringing life *to* the horse. The squirm may have been automatic, but the realization, created through counter casting, that three puppeteers can work together, breathe together, to lend their life to an inanimate object, that is what shifted my thinking. What and where is life? In the rehearsed ecosystem of the puppet operated by three men, life is when they are all working together; individuality is suspended. Basil Jones explains the magic of the puppets in this way: "Puppets always have to try to be alive. It's their kind of, Ur-story, onstage, that desperation to live." Adrian Kohler then added, "Yeah, it's basically a dead object, as you can see, but it only lives because you make it. An actor struggles to die onstage, and a puppet has to struggle to live, and in a way that's a metaphor for life."[27] The puppets cannot struggle alone, of course, but spread out over the work and effort of the system, life is possible. Squirming with the audience at the pain of a non-horse, the bounds between myself and the other spectators dissolved temporarily, and I could see the possibilities of a networked self.

An Extended Self

A networked self is plastic, changeable, more like the current research on the brain than the idea of individual, semiperme-able cells that was so popular in medical and literary research of the nineteenth century. This is particularly salient in light of research in cognitive science on extended and distributed cognition. Extended cognition is the theory that thinking expands beyond the "skin and skull."[28] Thinking is what happens between humans and their environmental tools, connecting seemingly discreet units (brain, hand, iPhone, etc.) into a cognizing system. If our environment becomes part of the cognitive act, we must extend what and where we imagine as the "mind." Distributed cognition, on the other hand, is a way of thinking about all cognition. According to Edwin Hutchins, "Distributed cognition begins with the assumption that all instances of cognition can be seen as emerging from distributed processes."[29] The process whereby a group of people launch a space shuttle or put on *Romeo and Juliet*, for example, can be seen as a distributed process where cognition is the result: the shuttle launch is successful, the play goes on. The value for theater and performance scholars lies not in which of these theories ultimately persuades the most scholars or scientists, the value lies in how we might rethink our categories of research.

We can use the metaphor of casting to put pressure on the idea of the self. In a recent promotional video for *The Atlantic*, actor Michael K. Williams wondered aloud whether or not he is being "typecast." Suddenly, there was another Michael K. Williams, dressed as a different character, sitting with him, debating him about the philosophical meaning of "playing" a character. Then a third Williams was there, dressed as Omar—his famous character from the HBO series *The Wire*—insisting that "this metaphor is bullshit. I think you are always going to be playing some version of Mike" but then each of the "versions" he listed contained the word "gangsta" before it, suggesting that there's only so far from racist typecasting Williams can get.[30] Through this counter casting though—staging several different Michael K. Williams characters at the same time—the viewer must see and question her protocols of casting, of building characters. I perceived a version of this "counter casting" during the Women's Marches in January 2017 when, through the connective tissue of the "pussy hats," women—and men—refused the part they were handed. We were not individuals, we were a united flock or swarm, held together by a common reaction to Trump's reference to women's "parts." Counter casting, refusing the individual parts we are asked to play and perceiving and playing new roles, is not just political; it's a reflection of contemporary scientific theories on extended cognition and the self.

There's a photograph of me as a toddler crying during a family portrait: the 1970s-dressed parents sit on chairs in a row, smiling broadly, and their daughter, well-dressed but pucker-faced, ruins the shot. This is the family photo that hung on our wall throughout my childhood, long after my brother came along and I stopped crying. Walking by it on the wall every day of my childhood, the photo called to me daily: "remember this. Remember there was a time when you had no power to choose your own clothes and your tears seemed to signal no danger." I came to believe that the photo remained on the wall because of a similar way that it hailed my parents as the persevering adults amid chaos; all of us used it to characterize the others. The cells that made up those people however, are long gone. I have nothing tangible in common with that girl. We do not share memories—not that memories are tangible anyway. They are not movies from the past but neural patterns, and they don't remain stable over time. The DNA that is in charge of making my replacement cells as I move from this Amy to another Amy is the same, but even it can be adjusted and affected by environment. However I may "cast" myself as some stable being with a relatively consistent personality, this idea is a fiction that holds me together; the fiction that I'm singular and isolated.

Not only do we not have some stable, essential self, we aren't even mostly "ourselves." It is now estimated that only 10 percent of the cells in and on our body contain our DNA. Close to 90 percent of the cells in and on "our" bodies belong to bacteria. In order to remain convinced of my identity, I have to block out recognition of the majority of what constitutes "me" (which is also always in flux) and hold together a carefully constructed network of memories and impressions to come up with a blend that I believe is "me." That is the definition of what a character is, the same way that Hamlet played by Olivier is a character or Lincoln played by Day-Lewis is a character. I am not the same person I was ten years ago in most of the ways that count: my cells have changed, my memories have changed, and my knowledge has changed. I create a narrative that serves as a frame within which I can hold this set of spaces together. It is precarious and it is precious. As bioethicist Rosamond Rhodes explains, "In the sense that our physical bodies and the space occupied by our microbiome are hard to delineate, and that the human microbiome genome cannot be entirely separated from the human genome, we are coexistent rather than independent beings."[31] What Rhodes suggests is a radical rethinking of our selves: from "independent" to "coexistent." This counter casting encourages me to think about "us" rather than about "me." What if each of the different kinds of bacteria in our bodies was competing for world domination and I, you, all of us, were just the battlefields on which they fight? Theater allows us to stage and thus contemplate the world around us. Casting is the creative and performative act that compresses and makes sense of the moving, living conspecifics we share the world with. Like that murmuration of starlings I started the book with, I can be us. I can refuse the character narrative.

Notes

Introduction

1. Andrea Peterson, "The Switch: The Sony Pictures Hack, Explained," the *Washington Post*, December 18, 2014, accessed December 2, 2016, https://www.washingtonpost.com/news/the-switch/wp/2014/12/18/the-sony-pictures-hack-explained/?utm_term=.95f9529ac692

2. "Is There Any Lighthearted News?" *The Rush Limbaugh Show*, December 23, 2014, accessed November 22, 2016, http://www.rushlimbaugh.com/daily/2014/12/23/is_there_any_lighthearted_news

3. Both Angela Pao and Brandi Wilkins Catanese offer important arguments about race and casting that I will take up more completely in chapter 3. See Angela C. Pao, *No Safe Spaces: Re-Casting Race, Ethnicity, and Nationality in American Theater* (Ann Arbor: University of Michigan Press, 2010); and Brandi Wilkins Catanese, *The Problem of the Color[Blind]: Racial Transgression and the Politics of Black Performance* (Ann Arbor: University of Michigan Press, 2011).

4. Robin Ross, "Rush Limbaugh Condemns Idris Elba as the Next Bond Because He's Black," *TV Guide, Today's News: Our Take*, December 25, 2014, accessed January 6, 2014, http://www.tvguide.com/news/rush-limbaugh-idris-elba-1091288/

The *TV Guide* article does point out that "while the first Bond was played by the Scottish Sean Connery, Roger Moore is English and Pierce Brosnan is Irish, something Limbaugh clearly forgot." Limbaugh's comments, not surprisingly, became noteworthy themselves. He responded to his critics on his show on January 4, 2015, by insisting he is not racist but still views the casting choice coming from "this girl Amy Pascal" as evidence of political pressure, not creativity.

5. Pao, *No Safe Spaces*, 127.

6. Wade Goodwyn, "Former Texas Gov. Rick Perry Launches Second Presidential Run," *All Things Considered*, NPR, June 4, 2015, 4:33 p.m. EST.

7. Brandi Wilkins Catanese, *The Problem of the Color[blind]: Racial Trans-*

gression and the Politics of Black Performance (Ann Arbor: University of Michigan Press, 2011), 20–22.

8. See "character, n." *OED Online*.

9. Lisa A. Freeman, *Character's Theater: Genre and Identity on the Eighteenth-Century English Stage* (Philadelphia: University of Pennsylvania Press, 2002), 8.

10. Ibid., 36.

11. Ibid., 28–29.

12. Ibid., 31.

13. Bert O. States, "The Anatomy of Dramatic Character," *Theatre Journal* 37, no. 1 (1985): 86–101.

14. I have articulated some of these ideas elsewhere. For an adaptation of these ideas to Shakespeare, see Amy Cook, "King of Shadows: Early Modern Characters and Actors," in *Shakespeare and Consciousness*, eds. Paul Budra and Clifford Werrier (New York: Palgrave Macmillan, 2016).

15. Bert States, *Hamlet and the Concept of Character* (Baltimore, MD: Johns Hopkins University Press, 1992), xiv.

16. Ibid., 18.

17. Blakey Vermeule, *Why Do We Care about Literary Characters?* (Baltimore, MD: Johns Hopkins University Press, 2009), esp. chapter 2.

18. The theory of mind (ToM) came from attempting to understand the problem of other minds: How do we understand that others can hold false beliefs, that others can think and feel different from us? Simon Baron-Cohen attributes autism to a deficiency in one's ToM; Simon Baron-Cohen, *Mindblindness: An Essay on Autism and Theory of Mind* (Cambridge, MA: MIT Press, 1995). The theory of mind is generally studied through a number of tests. An example is the "false-belief" task, in which two children are told a story about a hidden marble (or candy). Both children see where the object is hidden. One child leaves the room and the other child moves the object from where it was when the first child was in the room. The second child is then asked where the first child (the one who was out of the room when the object was moved) will look for the object. The second child passes or fails based on whether he or she can perceive that the first child will have different ideas from him or herself about where the object is. See Alvin Goldman, "Imitation, Mind Reading, and Simulation," in *Perspectives on Imitation II*, eds. S. Hurley and N. Chater (Cambridge, MA: MIT Press, 2005).

19. Lisa Zunshine, "Theory of Mind and Experimental Representations of Fictional Consciousness," *Narrative* 11, no. 3 (2003): 270–91, esp. 271. See

also Lisa Zunshine, *Why We Read Fiction: Theory of Mind and the Novel* (Columbus: Ohio State University Press, 2006).

20. While I find Zunshine's reading of Woolf incredibly persuasive and I agree about the power of serially embedded mental states in the perception of fiction, I am skeptical of theory of mind applications in literary and theater studies. There seems to be a divide among those of us who use cognitive science research to understand the humanities between theory of mind and more embodied approaches. As David Herman recently articulated at the second annual Cognitive Futures Conference in Durham, UK, theory of mind suggests that we generate mental representations (of some kind or another) about the mental states of others and that this can reify the Cartesian dualism that many cognitive scientists have been trying to escape. Mental representations suggest a process or image in the mind and then a mental process of assessing that representation. This evokes an infinite regress of representation and assessor—something for which there is not yet any evidence. Further, as Barbara Dancygier pointed out at the same conference, the idea of theory of mind comes from psychological false-belief tests and do not necessarily support the kind of mental-state reasoning that fiction encourages.

21. "Character-building" under "Character" in the *OED Online*.

22. "Character building experience," *Urban Dictionary*, accessed February 18, 2016. http://www.urbandictionary.com/define.php?term=character+building+experience

23. Quoted in Rob Kendt, *How They Cast It: An Insider's Look at Film and Television Casting* (Los Angeles: Lone Eagle Publishing, 2005), 159.

24. Rob Kendt, *How They Cast It: An Insider's Look at Film and Television Casting* (Los Angeles: Lone Eagle Publishing, 2005), 126.

25. Ibid., 120.

26. Ibid.

27. Marvin Carlson, *The Haunted Stage: The Theatre as Memory Machine* (Ann Arbor: University of Michigan Press, 2001), 9.

28. Tiffany Stern, *Making Shakespeare: From Stage to Page* (London: Routledge, 2004), 26.

29. Carlson, *The Haunted Stage*, 8.

30. Ibid., 166.

31. Ibid.

32. There are many who argue that there should be an Oscar for Best Casting. Perhaps because the first casting director, Marion Dougherty—who cast *Midnight Cowboy* and *Slaughterhouse-Five*, among many others—was a

woman, the position is viewed less centrally than Director of Photography. See *Casting By*, by Tom Donahue, HBO Documentaries, 2013.

33. Michael Quinn, "Celebrity and the Semiotics of Acting," *New Theatre Quarterly* 22 (1990): 154.

34. Joseph Roach, *It* (Ann Arbor: University of Michigan Press, 2007).

35. Joseph Roach, *Cities of the Dead: Circum-Atlantic Performance* (New York: Columbia University Press, 1996), 2.

36. Ibid., 36.

37. Ibid., 80. Citing *George Farquhar, Works*, ed. Shirley Strum Kenny, vol. 2. (Oxford Clarendon, 1988), 384.

38. This is true to some degree when an actor plays a part in a movie that was first a book, though in that case there is no physical body of the "original," just assumptions in the readers' minds. When actors play real people—such as Margaret Thatcher or Ray Charles or Richard Nixon—part of the performance is the virtuosity with which the actor brings to life a figure we know. Perhaps this is why these actors are so often nominated for Academy Awards. I will speak more about this in chapter 3.

39. Joseph A. Boone and Nancy J. Vickers, "Introduction: Celebrity Rites," *PMLA* 126, no. 4 (2011): 902. Boone and Vickers quoted Douglas Kellner, "Celebrity Diplomacy, Spectacle and Barack Obama," *Celebrity Studies* 1, no. 1 (2010): 121.

40. George Lakoff and Rafael Núñez, *Where Mathematics Come From: How the Embodied Mind Brings Mathematics Into Being* (New York: Basic Books, 2000).

41. George Lakoff and Mark Johnson, *Philosophy in the Flesh: The Embodied Mind and Its Challenge to Western Thought* (New York: Basic Books, 1999), 463.

42. Rolf A. Zwaan, Robert A. Stanfield, and Richard H. Yaxley, "Language Comprehenders Mentally Represent the Shapes of Objects," *Psychological Science*, 13, no. 2 (2002): 168–71.

43. Benjamin K. Bergen, *Louder Than Words: The New Science of How the Mind Makes Meaning* (New York: Basic, 2012), 57.

44. David Robson, "Kiki or Bouba? In Search of Language's Missing Link," *New Scientist* 2821, August 17, 2011, accessed July 8, 2015, http://www.newscientist.com/article/mg21128211.600-kiki-or-bouba-in-search-of-languages-missing-link.html?full=true&print=true#.VZ1Q_01VhHw

45. Raymond W. Gibbs Jr., *Embodiment and Cognitive Science* (New York: Cambridge University Press, 2005), 9.

46. A growing number of books are using embodied cognition to think with and through questions of art and the humanities. Some of these in-

fluential books are Rhonda Blair and Amy Cook, eds., *Theatre, Cognition Performance: Language, Bodies, Ecology* (New York: Methuen, 2016); Guillemette Bolens, *The Style of Gestures: Embodiment and Cognition in Literary Narrative* (Baltimore, MD: Johns Hopkins University Press, 2012); John Lutterbie, *Toward a General Theory of Acting* (New York: Palgrave Macmillan, 2011); Rhonda Blair, *The Actor, Image, and Action: Acting and Cognitive Neuroscience* (New York: Routledge, 2008); Barbara Dancygier, *The Language of Stories* (Cambridge, UK: Cambridge University Press, 2012); Bruce McConachie, *Engaging Audiences: A Cognitive Approach to Spectating in the Theatre* (New York: Palgrave Macmillan, 2008); Evelyn Tribble, *Cognition in the Globe: Attention and Memory in Shakespeare's Theatre* (New York, Palgrave, 2011); Naomi Rokotnitz, *Trusting Performance* (New York: Palgrave Macmillan, 2011); and Nicola Shaughnessy, ed., *Affective Performance and Cognitive Science: Body, Brain and Being* (London: Methuen, 2013).

47. Benjamin Bergen, *Louder Than Words* (New York: Basic, 2012), 79–80.

48. Arthur M. Glenberg, Marc Sato, Luigi Cattaneo, Lucia Riggio, Daniele Palumbo, Giovanni Buccino, "Processing Abstract Language Modulates Motor System Activity," *Quarterly Journal of Experimental Psychology* 61, no. 6 (2008): 905–19.

49. George Lakoff and Mark Johnson, *Metaphors We Live By* (Chicago: University of Chicago Press, 1980); and George Lakoff and Mark Turner, *More Than Cool Reason: A Field Guide to Poetic Metaphor* (Chicago: University of Chicago Press, 1989).

50. On mental spaces, see Gilles Fauconnier, *Mental Spaces: Aspects of Meaning Construction in Natural Language* (Cambridge: Cambridge University Press, 1985). For blending theory, see Gilles Fauconnier and Mark Turner, *The Way We Think: Conceptual Blending and the Mind's Hidden Complexities* (New York: Basic Books, 2002).

51. Fauconnier and Turner, *The Way We Think*, 16.

52. Fauconnier and Eve Sweetser, "Foreword," *Mental Spaces: Aspects of Meaning Construction in Natural Language*, 2nd ed. (Cambridge, UK: Cambridge University Press, 1994), x.

53. Ibid., 17–18.

54. I. A. Richards, *The Philosophy of Rhetoric* (New York: Oxford University Press, 1936), 96.

55. This is a 2001 advertisement for the Education Excellence Partnership copied in Fauconnier and Turner, *The Way We Think*, 67.

56. Gilles Fauconnier, "Compression and Emergent Structure," *Language and Linguistics* 6, no. 4 (2005): 534.

57. Ibid.

58. An argument could be made that the names in the script seem to call for children but do not require them. I will talk more about names in chapter 2.

59. Fauconnier and Turner, *The Way We Think*, 266–67.

60. Ibid.

61. For more on this see Amy Cook, "Staging Nothing: *Hamlet* and Cognitive Science," *SubStance* 35, no. 2, 2006; Bruce McConachie, *Engaging Audiences: A Cognitive Approach to Spectating in the Theatre* (New York, Basingstoke and London: Palgrave Macmillan, 2008); and Richard J. Gerrig, *Experiencing Narrative Worlds: On the Psychological Activities of Reading*, (New Haven, CT: Yale University Press, 1993).

62. McConachie, *Engaging Audiences*, 48.

63. Mark Turner, *The Origin of Ideas: Blending, Creativity, & The Human Spark* (Oxford, UK: Oxford University Press, 2014), 8.

64. More than other characters in Shakespeare, Henry has taken on different roles. He was "Hal" in the two parts of *Henry IV* (plays that were about him but were named for his father), a riotous youth who offers this explanation for his rejection of his friend and comrade, Falstaff: "Presume not that I am the thing I was, / For God doth know, so shall the world perceive, / That I have turn'd away my former self; / So will I those that kept me company" (5.5.56–59) and is now King Henry V. His title finally fits the title of the play he is in, but it defines him much the way the Chorus defines the ciphers: he is a king because he is the fifth in a line of Henrys. For more on Henry V and conceptual blending theory, see Cook, "The Narrative of Nothing: The Mathematical Blends of Narrator and Hero in Shakespeare's *Henry V*," *Blending and the Study of Narrative*, eds. Ralf Schneider and Marcus Hartner (Berlin: de Gruyter, 2012).

65. See F. Elizabeth Hart, "Review: The View of Where We've Been and Where We'd Like to Go," *College Literature: Cognitive Shakespeare: Criticism and Theory in the Age of Neuroscience* 33, no. 1 (2006): 233.

66. For approaches to literature that integrate research from cognitive linguistics, see Mary Crane, *Shakespeare's Brain: Reading with Cognitive Theory* (Princeton, NJ: Princeton University Press, 2001); Mary Crane and Alan Richardson, "Literary Studies and Cognitive Science: Toward a New Interdisciplinarity," *Mosaic* 32, no. 2 (1999): 124–40, Dancygier, *The Language of Stories*; Donald C. Freeman, "Othello and the 'Ocular Proof,'" *The Shakespearean International Yearbook*, vol. 4 (Aldershot: Ashgate Publishing, 2004), 56–71; Patrick Colm Hogan, *Cognitive Science, Literature, and the Arts: A Guide for Humanists* (New York: Routledge, 2003); Ellen Spolsky,

Word vs Image: Cognitive Hunger in Shakespeare's England (Basingstoke: Palgrave Macmillan, 2007); Eve Sweetser, "Whose Rhyme Is Whose Reason? Sound and Sense in *Cyrano de Bergerac*," *Language and Linguistics* 15, no. 1 (2006): 29–54; and Mark Turner, *The Literary Mind: The Origins of Thought and Language* (Oxford: Oxford University Press, 1996).

67. For applications of cognitive science research to theater and performance studies, see Rhonda Blair, *The Actor, Image, and Action: Acting and Cognitive Neuroscience* (New York: Routledge, 2008); Cook, *Shakespearean Neuroplay* (New York: Palgrave Macmillan, 2010); Rokotnitz, *Trusting Performance* (New York: Palgrave Macmillan, 2011); McConachie, *Engaging Audiences* (New York, Basingstoke and London: Palgrave Macmillan, 2008); Rick Kemp, *Embodied Acting: What Neuroscience Tells Us about Performance* (New York: Routledge, 2012); and John Lutterbie, *Toward a General Theory of Acting* (New York: Palgrave Macmillan, 2011).

68. Brian MacWhinney, "The Emergence of Grammar from Perspective," in *Grounding Cognition: The Role of Perception and Action in Memory, Language and Thinking*, eds. Diane Pecher and Rolf A. Zwaan (Cambridge: Cambridge University Press, 2005), 203.

69. Diane Pecher and Rolf A. Zwaan, "Introduction to Grounding Cognition: The Role of Perception and Action in Memory, Language and Thinking," in *Grounding Cognition: The Role of Perception and Action in Memory, Language and Thinking*, eds. Diane Pecher and Rolf A. Zwaan (Cambridge: Cambridge University Press, 2005), 2.

70. Unless we have prosopagnosia, but more on that in the next chapter.

71. Some of this problem might alter or be reformulated if cognition is simulated instead of representational, but the basic challenges posed by this problem remain, as does the importance of categorization.

72. James J. Gibson, *The Ecological Approach to Visual Perception* (Boston: Houghton-Mifflin, 1979).

73. Eleanor Rosch, "Principles of Categorization," in *Foundations of Cognitive Psychology (Core Readings)*, ed. Daniel J. Levitin (Cambridge: MIT Press, 2002), 251.

74. Lakoff, *Women, Fire, and Dangerous Things: What Categories Reveal about the Mind* (Chicago: University of Chicago Press, 1987), 93.

75. Ibid., 95.

76. There is a strange gap between the scholarship of film and theater/performance studies in this area, and this will not be the place to address it. One problem, for me, is that a lot of early cognitive film studies is disembodied. An exception to this is Maarten Coëgnarts and Peter Kravanja,

eds., *Embodied Cognition and Cinema* (Leuven, Belgium: Leuven University Press, 2015).

Chapter 1

1. This worked partially to counter online discussion about whether or not Ledger was the right choice to play the Joker. Thinking about Ledger's previous roles as "closeted gay cowboy Ennis Del Mar in *Brokeback Mountain* the year before, and bad boy Patrick Verona in the teen movie *10 Things I Hate About You*," fans took to the internet to say things like "I won't be able to watch it. I'll keep expecting him to have sex with Batman." With his past films as a guide, these anticipatory critics composed a character capable of inventing new storylines—kissing Batman, being described as "cute." See Alice Vincent, "In 2006, nobody wanted Heath Ledger to play the Joker," *The Telegraph*, May 26, 2016, accessed February 20, 2017, http://www.tele graph.co.uk/films/2016/04/14/in-2006-nobody-wanted-heath-ledger-to-play-the-joker/

2. An image of this popular Internet meme from 2014 can be found at weheartit.com/entry/group/28078589

3. Mark Johnson, *The Meaning of the Body: Aesthetics of Human Understanding* (Chicago: University of Chicago Press, 2007), 132.

4. Gilles Fauconnier and Mark Turner, *The Way We Think: Conceptual Blending and the Mind's Hidden Complexities* (New York: Basic Books, 2002), 323–24.

5. Amy Cook, *Shakespearean Neuroplay: Reinvigorating the Study of Dramatic Texts and Performance through Cognitive Science* (New York: Palgrave Macmillan, 2010), 112.

6. I am grateful to Scott Magelssen and his graduate students at the University of Washington for pointing out the efficacy of casting Bill Murray in this film.

7. Murray did play Herman Blume in Wes Anderson's *Rushmore* in 1998, but this could still be considered a comic part in a serious film or a serious part in a comic film—like *The Royal Tenenbaums*, which followed in 2001. It was after *Rushmore* that Murray's personas began to shift; he played Bob Harris in *Lost in Translation* and Don Johnston in Jim Jarmusch's *Broken Flowers* (2005). Casting Bill Murray in 1991 (in *What about Bob?*) is very different from casting him in 2003 (in *Lost in Translation*), and not just because of the age difference; through the roles he accepted, Murray began to

reshape both the characters he played and the associations people brought to the roles he played.

8. Lisa S. Starks, "The Displaced Body of Desire: Sexuality in Kenneth Branagh's *Hamlet*" in *Shakespeare and Appropriation*, eds. Christy Desmet and Robert Sawyer (London: Routledge, 1999), 171.

9. Barbara Hodgdon, "Replicating Richard: Body Doubles, Body Politics," *Theatre Journal* 50, no. 2 (1998): 207. Keir Elam, "In What Chapter of His Bosom? Reading Shakespeare's Bodies" in *Alternative Shakespeares, vol. 2*, ed. Terence Hawkes (London: Routledge, 1996), 163.

10. Ibid., 208.

11. Ibid., 217.

12. Ibid., 220.

13. Judith Butler, *Excitable Speech: A Politics of the Performative* (New York: Routledge, 1997), 122, quoted in Hodgdon, "Replicating Richard," 221.

14. Though I agree about the power of performance to rehearse and create change, Butler's work, as Bruce McConachie and F. Elizabeth Hart have argued, relies on a structuralist assumption of language comprehension. As Hart points out, "both deconstruction and materialist studies have internalized basic formalist assumptions about the operations of language that are indigenous to linguistic structuralism." See Hart, "Matter, System, and Early Modern Studies: Outlines for a Materialist Linguistics," *Configurations* 6, no. 3 (1998): 313–14. Eve Sweetser brilliantly explains how Butler's notion of the performative fails to make sense within a cognitive framework, while also arguing that the idea that ideas can be operational, or performative, through acts has a cognitive corollary in conceptual blending theory. See Sweetser, "Blended Spaces and Performativity," *Cognitive Linguistics* 11, nos. 3/4 (2000). For a strong argument for the integration of the sciences into the humanities, see Bruce McConachie, "Falsifiable Theories for Theatre and Performance Studies," *Theatre Journal* 59, no. 4 (2007): 553–77.

15. The trailer can be seen at "Titus–Trailer," YouTube video, https://www.youtube.com/watch?v=usD_8_-tfvY

16. Samuel Crowl, *Shakespeare at the Cineplex: The Kenneth Branagh Era* (Athens: University of Ohio Press, 2003), 208.

17. Janet Maslin, "More Things in 'Hamlet' than Are Dreamt of in Other Adaptations," *New York Times*, December 25, 1996. Accessed December 12, 2016, http://www.nytimes.com/movie/review?res=9B0CE5D91E31F936A15751C1A960958260&pagewanted=print

18. Shakespeare also used casting to point metatheatrically beyond the text. When Hamlet asks Polonius about his acting past and Polonius re-

ports, "I did enact Julius Caesar. I was killed i' th' Capitol. Brutus killed me," Hamlet responds, "It was a brute part of him to kill so capital a calf there" (3.2.101–104). Arden editor Harold Jenkins notes that the original actors of Hamlet and Polonius probably played Caesar and Brutus in the 1599 production of *Julius Caesar,* and therefore, through their characters, both actors are gesturing to another stage relationship they shared. Tiffany Stern's analysis of the *Julius Caesar* conversation in *Hamlet* points out the particularity of the theatrical reference: Shakespeare could have had Polonius refer to a role not included in the plays of his own writing (e.g., Polonius could have played Herod), but then Shakespeare would have been referring to another text, not just another performance. If, as is assumed, Burbage played Hamlet in 1600 and he played Brutus the year before, Polonius is simultaneously speaking to both Hamlet and Burbage. Burbage, onstage in 1600 as Hamlet, cannot completely slip the roles he has played in the past. See Stern, *Making Shakespeare: From Stage to Page* (London: Routledge, 2004), 74, and Jenkins, ed., *Hamlet* (Surrey, UK: Arden Shakespeare, 1982): 294.

19. In fact, I might argue that the audience of Shakespeare's time had the same experience: that character was played by the clown. The sight of the clown talking back to the prince in the graveyard, of tossing about skulls, is funny in and of itself. For those who did not follow the jesting and word play—though I do not think it would have been difficult for the groundlings in Shakespeare's theater—it might have been enough to perceive that there is comic levity at this point in the play.

20. Bert States might call this the "collaborative mode," wherein the actor "aligns the audience empathetically with his critical self, not the self he is portraying." States, *Hamlet and the Concept of Character* (Baltimore, MD: Johns Hopkins University Press, 1992), 31.

21. In an interview Ben Stiller gave for *The Spinning Image,* the interviewer asks, "Was it always your intention to have Spider Man and Iron Man making out (in Robert Downey Jr.'s fake trailer in the movie)?" The question alludes to the fact that the actor who played Spider Man (Tobey Maguire) has a cameo kissing Robert Downey Jr., who plays Iron Man in other movies but also plays Kirk Lazarus, Method actor, in *Tropic Thunder.* Ben Stiller's response, after laughing, is: "No that totally just happened! Actually Tobey was a last minute replacement for that, he did us a big favour. It turned out to be one of those things where the replacement ends up being better than the first choice. Afterwards, when I realised it was Iron Man and Spider-man making out, that was just even better!" The blend between actor and character is such that an actor can remain permanently linked

to the character, allowing such impossibilities as Spider Man kissing Iron Man. Graeme Clark, "*Tropic Thunder:* The Stars Speak," *The Spinning Image*, accessed November 28, 2016, http://www.thespinningimage.co.uk/article/displayarticle.asp?articleid=98

22. John Macnamara, *Names for Things: A Study of Human Learning* (Cambridge, MA: MIT Press, 1984), 31.

23. Raphael Lyne, *Shakespeare, Rhetoric and Cognition* (Cambridge, UK: Cambridge University Press, 2011), 125–26.

24. Ibid., 127.

25. Murray J. Levith, *What's in Shakespeare's Names?* (Hamden, CT: Archon Books, 1978), 19.

26. Ibid., 20, 21.

27. Ibid., 44.

28. Jonathan Bate, ed., *Titus Andronicus* (London: Routledge, 1995), 18.

29. Michael Ramscar, Asha Halima Smith, Melody Dye, Richard Futrell, Peter Hendrix, Harald Baayen, and Rebecca Starr, "The 'Universal' Structure of Name Grammars and the Impact of Social Engineering on the Evolution of Natural Information Systems," in *Proceedings of the 35th Meeting of the Cognitive Science Society*, eds. M. Knauff, M. Pauen, N. Sebanz, and I. Wachsmuth (Berlin: Cognitive Science Society, 2013), 3246–47.

30. In 2009, a bakery in New Jersey refused to decorate a birthday cake for young Adolph Hitler Campbell. Katie Steinmetz, "From Messiah to Hitler, What You Can and Cannot Name Your Child: A Judge's Order Calls Attention to Rules Governing Baby Names," *Time*, August 12, 2013, accessed February 23, 2015, http://nation.time.com/2013/08/12/from-messiah-to-hitler-what-you-can-and-cannot-name-your-child/

31. Ben Popken, "Royal Baby Name? 500-to-1 Odds on 'Macbeth'" *Today*, September 9, 2014, accessed February 19, 2017, http://www.today.com/money/royal-baby-name-500-1-odds-macbeth-1D80137605

32. Evelyn Tribble, *Cognition in the Globe: Attention and Memory in Shakespeare's Theatre* (New York: Palgrave Macmillan, 2011), 20, Tribble's italics.

33. Richard J. Gerrig and David N. Rapp, "Psychological Processes Underlying Literary Impact," *Poetics Today* 25, no. 2 (2004): 272.

34. Ibid., 272–73.

35. Richard J. Gerrig and David W. Allbritton, "The Construction of Literary Character: A View from Cognitive Psychology," *Style* 24 (Fall 1990): 3.

36. Suzanne Keen, "Readers' Temperaments and Fictional Character," *New Literary History* 42, no. 2 (2011): 295.

37. Ibid., 310.

38. See, for example, the discussion in *Trends in Cognitive Sciences:* Leon de Bruin and Shaun Gallagher, "Embodied Simulation, an Unproductive Explanation: Comment on Gallese and Sinigaglia," *Trends in Cognitive Sciences* 16, no. 2 (February 2012): 98–99, and Vittorio Gallese and Corrado Sinigaglia, "Letter: Response to de Bruin and Gallagher: Embodied Simulation as Reuse Is a Productive Explanation of a Basic Form of Mind-Reading," *Trends in Cognitive Sciences* 16, no. 2 (February 2012): 99–100.

39. Andy Clark, *Supersizing the Mind: Embodiment, Action, and Cognitive Extension* (New York: Oxford University Press, 2008), 46.

40. For an analysis of the conceptual integration network involved in Hamlet's "mirror held up to nature," including a discussion of the personification of Virtue at work in the text, see Cook, *Shakespearean Neuroplay.*

41. I'm using anchor here as Edwin Hutchins does in his important book, *Cognition in the Wild* (Cambridge, MA: MIT Press, 1995).

42. "Prosopagnosia," YouTube video, accessed February 3, 2015, https://www.youtube.com/watch?v=vwCrxomPbtY

43. Richard Russell, Brad Duchaine, and Ken Nakayama, "Super-Recognizers: People with Extraordinary Face Recognition Ability," *Psychonomic Bulletin & Review* 16, no. 2 (2009): 252–57, accessed June 26, 2015.

44. Ibid.

45. Ibid.

46. Ibid.

47. V. S. Ramachandran and Sandra Blakeslee, *Phantoms in the Brain: Probing the Mysteries of the Human Mind* (New York: Quill William Morrow, 1998), 164.

48. Ibid., 166.

49. Hadyn D. Ellis and Michael B. Lewis, "Capgras Delusion: A Window on Face Recognition," *Trends in Cognitive Sciences* 5, no. 4 (2001): 156.

50. Robert Krulwich, "Neuroscientists Battle Furiously over Jennifer Aniston," *Krulwich Wonders: Robert Krulwich on Science*, March 30, 2012, accessed November 29, 2016, http://www.npr.org/sections/krulwich/2012/03/30/149685880/neuroscientists-battle-furiously-over-jennifer-aniston

51. Rodrigo Quian Quiroga, "Searching for the Jennifer Aniston Neuron," *Scientific American*, February 1, 2013, http://www.scientificamerican.com/article/brain-cells-searching-for-jennifer-aniston-neuron/, accessed April 20, 2015. It is an excerpt from Quiroga's book, *Borges and Memory: Encounters with the Human Brain* (Cambridge, MA: MIT Press, 2013).

52. Rodrigo Quian Quiroga, Itzhak Fried, and Christof Koch, "Brain Cells for Grandmother," *Scientific American*, February 2013, 3135. Accessed April

20, 2015. https://www2.le.ac.uk/centres/csn/publications-1/Publications/scientificamerican0213–30.pdf

53. John Emigh, "Minding Bodies: Demons, Masks, Archetypes, and the Limits of Culture," *Journal of Dramatic Theory and Criticism* 25, no. 2 (2011): 125.

54. Richard Maxwell, *Theater for Beginners* (New York: TCG, 2015), 53–54.

55. Emily Hodgson Anderson, "Celebrity Shylock," *PMLA* 126, no. 4 (2011): 937, 938.

Chapter 2

1. "Maggie Smith on the Pressures of Acting: 'You Want So Much to Get It Right,'" *Fresh Air*, February 23, 2016, http://www.npr.org/2016/02/23/467802382/maggie-smith-on-the-pressures-of-acting-you-want-so-much-to-get-it-right

2. Ibid.

3. Leo Braudy, *The Frenzy of Renown: Fame and Its History* (New York: Oxford University Press, 1986), 1071.

4. Ibid., 553.

5. Richard Dyer, *Heavenly Bodies: Film Stars and Society* (New York: St. Martin's Press, 1986), 8.

6. Sharon Marcus, "The Celebrity System circa 1879," unpublished talk (Indiana University, September 13, 2013), 23.

7. Marcus, "Salomé!! Sarah Bernhardt, Oscar Wilde, and the Drama of Celebrity," *PMLA* 126, no. 4 (2011): 1003–4.

8. Emily Hodgson Anderson, "Celebrity Shylock," *PMLA* 126, no. 4 (2011): 939, citing Lisa A. Freeman, *Character's Theater: Genre and Identity on the Eighteenth-Century English Stage* (Philadelphia: University of Pennsylvania Press, 2002), 936.

9. Linda Charnes, *Notorious Identity: Materializing the Subject in Shakespeare* (Cambridge, MA: Harvard University Press, 1993), 11.

10. Ibid., 9.

11. Joseph Roach, *It* (Ann Arbor: University of Michigan Press, 2007), 9.

12. Ben Brantley, "Threesome to Tantalize and Behold: Daniel Craig and Rachel Weisz Star in 'Betrayal' on Broadway," *New York Times*, October 27, 2013. Accessed December 26, 2016. http://www.nytimes.com/2013/10/28/theater/reviews/daniel-craig-and-rachel-weisz-star-in-betrayal-on-broadway.html

13. Tim Goodman, "Tim Goodman on James Gandolfini: 'You Couldn't Look Away From Him'" *The Hollywood Reporter*, posted at 6:08 p.m., June 19, 2013. Accessed January 8, 2015. http://www.hollywoodreporter.com/bastard-machine/james-gandolfini-death-sopranos-star-571900

14. Manohla Dargis, review of *Where the Wild Things Are* (2009), "Some of His Best Friends Are Beasts," *New York Times*, October 15, 2009. Accessed January 8, 2015. http://www.nytimes.com/2009/10/16/movies/16where.html?pagewanted=all&_r=0

15. It is worth noting that Sendak has not confused children with this story, despite the fact that the real world does not contain such wild things. We can refer to something in the world—a horse—or something not in the world—a unicorn—and be understood. This is possible in part because our language does not depend on correspondence between something out in the world and a word used to describe it. If it did, we could not speak of unicorns or utopias. Central to this ability is an alternative understanding of categories, an expanded role for metaphor, and the efficient and creative work of compression. Children are not bothered by the impossible or by nonsense; they are enriched by it. Mark Turner discusses a child's facility with these kinds of complicated blends in *The Literary Mind,* (New York: Oxford University Press, 1996) and *The Runaway Bunny* and specifically in Turner, "Double-Scope Stories," *Narrative Theory and the Cognitive Sciences*, ed. David Herman (CSLI, 2003), 17. I extend his example of *The Runaway Bunny* in *Shakespearean Neuroplay* (New York: Palgrave Macmillan, 2010), 12–13. For the influence of nonsense, see Benedict Carey, "How Nonsense Sharpens the Intellect," *New York Times*, October 5, 2009, accessed March 1, 2016, http://www.nytimes.com/2009/10/06/health/06mind.html?_r=0

16. "Designing the Creatures for 'Where the Wild Things Are,'" YouTube video, accessed February 4, 2015, https://www.youtube.com/watch?v=6QOBIGVCGpw

17. Joseph Roach, *It*, 9.

18. Emily Nussbaum, "Cheaper by the Dozen: Tatiana Maslany's Magnificent Sister Act, on 'Orphan Black,'" *The New Yorker*, April 28, 2014.

19. Ibid.

20. Lili Loofbourow, "The Many Faces of Tatiana Maslany," *New York Times Magazine*, April 2, 2015.

21. David Freedberg and Vittorio Gallese, "Motion, Emotion and Empathy in Esthetic Experience," *Trends in Cognitive Sciences*, 11, no. 5 (2007): 197.

22. See Lisa Zunshine, *Why We Read Fiction* (Columbus, OH: Ohio State University Press, 2006).

23. Mal Vincent, "Duvall Du Jour: Duvall, 'The Most Subtle of Actors,' Disappears into His Varied Characters," *Daily News* (Los Angeles), April 12, 1996.

24. Rick Kemp, *Embodied Acting: What Neuroscience Tells Us about Performance* (London: Routledge, 2012), 93. Italics in the original.

25. Ibid., 131.

26. Bert O. States, "The Actor's Presence: Three Phenomenal Modes," in *Acting (Re)Considered: A Theoretical and Practical Guide*, 2nd ed., ed. Phillip B. Zarrilli (London: Routledge, 2002), 25–26.

27. The video can be watched here: https://www.youtube.com/watch?v=ZyU213nhrh0, accessed January 2, 2017.

28. Ellen Terry, *Four Lectures on Shakespeare*, ed. Christopher St. John (London: Martin Hopkinson Ltd, 1932), 162.

29. Ibid., 163.

30. Joseph Roach, "It," *Theatre Journal* 56, no. 4, (Dec. 2004): 568.

31. Gregory Wakeman, "How Much Weight Was Carrie Fisher Asked to Lose for *Star Wars: The Force Awakens*" http://www.cinemablend.com/new/How-Much-Weight-Carrie-Fisher-Was-Asked-Lose-Star-Wars-Force-Awakens-97497.html, accessed January 2, 2017. See also, Heidi Hunter, "She Was TOLD to Lose 35 Pounds! Carrie Fisher Reveals She Had to Drop a Substantial Amount of Weight before Reprising Princess Leia Role in *Star Wars: Episode VII*," *Daily Mail*, May 16, 2014. http://www.dailymail.co.uk/tvshowbiz/article-2630644/She-TOLD-lose-35-pounds-Carrie-Fisher-reveals-Star-Wars-VII-dropped-substantial-weight.html#ixzz4UcOWjow7, accessed January 2, 2017.

32. Ryan Parker, "Carrie Fisher Responds to Criticism about Her Look in New 'Star Wars,'" *The Hollywood Reporter*, December 29, 2015. http://www.hollywoodreporter.com/news/carrie-fisher-responds-criticism-her-851448, accessed January 2, 2017.

33. Sue Bell, "The Force Awakens but What Happened to Carrie Fisher's Face?" Midlifexpress.com. http://midlifexpress.com/the-force-awakens-but-what-happened-to-carrie-fishers-face/, accessed January 2, 2017.

34. Toni Akindele, "The Comedian Took to Twitter When No Designer Would Dress Her for the Premiere of Her Upcoming *Ghostbusters* Reboot," *Essence*, June 29, 2016. http://www.essence.com/2016/06/29/leslie-jones-ghostbusters-designer-dress-discrimination, accessed January 2, 2017.

35. Angela C. Pao, *No Safe Spaces: Re-Casting Race, Ethnicity, and Nationality in American Theater* (Ann Arbor: University of Michigan Press, 2010), 26.

36. Ibid., 27.

37. Robert Brustein and August Wilson, "Subsidized Separatism: Responses to 'The Ground on Which I Stand,'" *American Theatre*, October 1996. http://www.americantheatre.org/1996/10/01/subsidized-separatism-responses-to-the-ground-on-which-i-stand/, accessed January 2, 2017. Both authors respond here to Wilson's Keynote Address to the Theatre Communications Group's Conference of June 1996.

38. Brandi Wilkins Catanese, *The Problem of the Color[blind]: Racial Transgression and the Politics of Black Performance* (Ann Arbor: University of Michigan Press, 2011), 21.

39. Ibid., 68

40. Ibid., 88.

41. Ibid., 91.

42. Ben Brantley, "Review: In 'Hamilton,' Lin-Manuel Miranda Forges Democracy through Rap," *New York Times*, February 16, 2015, accessed February 28, 2016, http://www.nytimes.com/2015/02/18/theater/review-in-hamilton-lin-manuel-miranda-forges-democracy-through-rap.html

43. Charles, McNulty, "Critic's Notebook: 'Hamilton's' Revolutionary Power Is in Its Hip-Hop Musical Numbers," *Los Angeles Times*, November 4, 2015, accessed February 28, 2016, http://www.latimes.com/entertainment/arts/la-ca-cm-hamilton-hip-hop-notebook-20151031-column.html

44. An "acting edition" of a play or musical is a version published specifically for licensed productions of the show. They will contain information regarding the original production and casting as well as direction from the playwright about show requirements, from setting information to casting stipulations. An acting edition is created when the author of the show—in this case Miranda—is no longer directly involved in production (as he is for the London and Chicago versions currently in production) but instead grants regional theatres, colleges, and high schools the right to perform his show.

45. Howard Sherman, "What Does 'Hamilton' Tell Us about Race in Casting?" December 3, 2015, accessed February 28, 2016, http://www.hesherman.com/2015/12/03/what-does-hamilton-tell-us-about-race-in-casting/

46. Laura Collins-Hughes, "Review: 'Awake and Sing!' a Depression-Era Family Drama," *New York Times*, July 20, 2015, accessed February 28, 2016,

http://www.nytimes.com/2015/07/21/theater/review-awake-and-sing-a-depression-era-family-drama.html

47. *Mule Bone*, by Langston Hughes and Zora Neale Hurston was written in 1930—five years before *Awake and Sing!*—and is not explicitly about racial issues either, despite being written by two African American writers. It is not considered a "classic," and it wasn't even produced until 1991. *Raisin in the Sun* (1959) by Lorraine Hansberry, on the other hand, is certainly considered a classic, but it is explicitly about issues of race.

48. Alexis Soloski, "She'll Play the Jewish Mother, and Wants Other Asian-Americans to Get the Best Parts, Too," *New York Times*, June 25, 2015, accessed February 28, 2016, http://www.nytimes.com/2015/06/28/theater/an-asian-american-theater-company-cuts-a-fresh-casting-trail.html

49. Katori Hall, "Playwright Reacts to the White Casting of MLK in *The Mountaintop*," *The Root*, November 9, 2015, accessed February 28, 2016, http://www.theroot.com/articles/culture/2015/11/the_white_version_of_mlk_in_the_mountaintop.html

50. Diep Tran, "On the Rights of Playwrights and White Tears: Lloyd Suh and Katori Hall Offer the Latest Teaching Moments in Race-Conscious Casting," *American Theatre*, November 16, 2015, accessed February 28, 2016, http://www.americantheatre.org/2015/11/16/on-the-rights-of-playwrights-and-white-tears/

51. August Wilson, "The Ground on Which I Stand," *Callaloo*, 20 no. 3 (1997): 497.

52. "What It's Really Like to Work in Hollywood* (*If You're Not a Straight White Man)," *New York Times*, February 24, 2016, accessed November 30, 2016, http://www.nytimes.com/interactive/2016/02/24/arts/hollywood-diversity-inclusion.html?_r=0

53. Catanese, *The Problem of the Color[blind]*, 9.

54. Ibid., 9–10.

55. Ayanna Thompson, *Passing Strange: Shakespeare, Race, and Contemporary America* (New York: Oxford University Press, 2011), 5.

56. Ayanna Thompson, "'Ay, There's the Rub': Race and Performance Studies," in *New Directions in Renaissance Drama and Performance Studies*, ed. Sarah Werner (London: Palgrave Macmillan, 2010), 189. Italics in the original.

57. Philip Auslander, *Performing Glam Rock: Gender and Theatricality in Popular Music* (Ann Arbor: University of Michigan Press, 2006), 39–40.

58. Ibid., 135.

59. Ibid., 138.

60. "Dr. Dre—Bitches Ain't Shit," YouTube video, https://www.youtube.com/watch?v=KUfzMDryA94 The full lyrics are at "Bitches Ain't Shit: Dr. Dre," *Genius*, http://genius.com/Dr-dre-bitches-aint-shit-lyrics

61. Some reviews point out that the song "throw[s]s heat Eazy-E's way," referring to the well-publicized legal and personal fight between Dr. Dre and Eazy-E after the breakup of N.W.A. In fact, the first "bitch" referred to in the song is Eazy-E. This does not decrease the misogyny so much as increase the "heat" thrown at Eazy-E, who is cast as nothing but a ho and a trick. Havelock Nelson, "Dr. Dre: The Chronic," *Rolling Stone*, March 18, 1993, accessed August 17, 2015, http://www.rollingstone.com/music/album reviews/the-chronic-19930318

62. Havelock Nelson, "The Chronic" Review, *Rolling Stone*, March 18, 1993. Accessed online August 17, 2015, http://www.rollingstone.com/music/album reviews/the-chronic-19930318

63. "Dr. Dre, 'The Chronic' at 20: Classic Track-By-Track Review," *Billboard*, December 15, 2012. Accessed August 17, 2015, http://www.billboard.com/articles/review/1537948/dr-dre-the-chronic-at-20-classic-track-by-track-review

64. Brent Staples, "The Politics of Gangsta Rap: A Music Celebrating Murder and Misogyny," Editorial Notebook. *New York Times*, August 27, 1993. Accessed August 17, 2015. http://www.nytimes.com/1993/08/27/opinion/editorial-notebook-the-politics-of-gangster-rap.html

65. Ibid.

66. Jon Pareles, "Critic's Notebook: Rappers Making Notoriety Pay Off," *New York Times*, October 31, 1995, accessed August 17, 2015, http://www.nytimes.com/1995/10/31/arts/critic-s-notebook-rappers-making-notoriety-pay-off.html

67. Pao, *No Safe Spaces*, 26.

68. Brent Staples, "The Politics of Gangsta Rap: A Music Celebrating Murder and Misogyny," *New York Times*, August 27, 1993. Accessed August 17, 2015.

69. "Ben Folds—Bitches Ain't Shit (Live)" YouTube video. Accessed August 17, 2015. https://www.youtube.com/watch?v=lxh2TRoef1Y

70. According to Marjorie Garber, when Cleopatra speaks of squeaking Cleopatras in the future, she is using the verb "to boy" to mean playing the boy's part, which "is to be anything but a man." Marjorie Garber, *Vested Interests: Cross-Dressing & Cultural Anxiety* (New York: Routledge, 1992), 89.

71. Ibid., 32.

72. Ibid., 90.

Chapter 3

1. Images of the *Pietá* can be found at http://stpetersbasilica.info/ Altars/Pieta/Pieta.htm.

2. Giorgio Vasari, *Lives of the Artists*, trans. George Bull (New York: Penguin, 1971).

3. Lawrence E. Williams and John A. Bargh, "Experiencing Physical Warmth Promotes Interpersonal Warmth," *Science* 322m, no.5901 (Oct. 24, 2008): 606–7.

4. David Kirsh and Paul Maglio, "On Distinguishing Epistemic from Pragmatic Action," *Cognitive Science* 18, no. 4 (1994): 513.

5. Philip Robbins and Murat Aydede, *The Cambridge Handbook of Situated Cognition* (New York: Cambridge University Press, 2009), 3.

6. Ibid.

7. Evelyn B. Tribble, *Cognition in the Globe: Attention and Memory in Shakespeare's Theatre* (New York: Palgrave Macmillan, 2011).

8. Bruce McConachie and F. Elizabeth Hart, *Performance and Cognition: Performance Studies and the Cognitive Turn* (London: Routledge, 2007).

9. Barbara Dancygier, "Multimodality and Theatre: Material Objects, Bodies and Language," in *Theatre, Performance and Cognition: Languages, Bodies and Ecologies*, eds. Rhonda Blair and Amy Cook (London: Methuen, 2016), 32.

10. Tom Stoppard, *Arcadia* (London: Faber and Faber, Inc., 1993), 15.

11. Dancygier, "Multimodality and Theatre: Material Objects, Bodies and Language," 26.

12. Evelyn Tribble and John Sutton, "Cognitive Ecology as a Framework for Shakespearean Studies," *Shakespeare Studies* 39 (2011): 94, 96.

13. Amy Cook, *Shakespearean Neuroplay*, 110–11. *Reinvigorating the Study of Dramatic Texts and Performance through Cognitive Science* (London: Palgrave Macmillan, 2010), 110–11.

14. Michael Billington, "Julius Caesar: Review," *The Guardian*, December 4, 2013, accessed May 31, 2016, https://www.theguardian.com/stage/2012/jun/07/julius-caesar-review

15. Ben Brantley, "Review: 'Henry IV,' Donmar Warehouse's All-Female

Version," *New York Times*, November 11, 2015, accessed May 31, 2016, http://
www.nytimes.com/2015/11/12/theater/review-henry-iv-donmar-ware
houses-all-female-version.html

16. *Taming of the Shrew,* The Public Theater's Shakespeare in the Park, dir.
Phyllida Lloyd. The Delacourte, NYC, May 28, 2016. Program, Director's
Notes.

17. Judy Gold as Gremio in *Taming of the Shrew*, The Public Theater's
Shakespeare in the Park, dir. Phyllida Lloyd. The Delacourte, NYC, May 28,
2016.

18. Eve Ensler, *The Vagina Monologues* (New York: Villard, 1998), 4.

19. Robert Simonson, "Off-Bway's *Vagina Monologues* Nets Stars a-
Plenty," *Playbill*, January 24, 2000.

20. James Barron, "Public Lives," *New York Times*, April 25, 2000, B2, accessed December 30, 2015, http://www.nytimes.com/2000/04/25/nyre-
gion/public-lives.html

21. Simonson, "Off-Bway's *Vagina Monologues* Nets Stars A-Plenty."

22. Jesse McKinley, "'Monologues' Making a Political Connection," *New
York Times*, April 21, 2000, B2, accessed December 30, 2015, http://www.
nytimes.com/2000/04/21/nyregion/monologues-making-a-political-
connection.html

23. Barron, "Public Lives."

24. Elisabeth Bumiller, "Giuliani's Wife Postpones Her Role in 'Monologues,' *New York Times, May 2, 2000, B1, accessed December 30, 2015,* http://
www.nytimes.com/2000/05/02/nyregion/giuliani-s-wife-postpones-her-
role-in-monologues.html

25. Elisabeth Bumiller "Mayor's Wife Begins Her Run in 'Monologues'
(Donna Hanover)," *New York Times*, October 18, 2000, B3, accessed December 30, 2015, http://www.nytimes.com/2000/10/18/nyregion/mayor-s-
wife-begins-her-run-in-monologues.html

26. Carol Martin and Anna Deavere Smith, "Anna Deavere Smith: The
Word Becomes You. An Interview," *TDR* 37, no. 4 (1993): 51.

27. On symptomatic versus surface reading, see Stephen Best and Sharon Marcus, "Surface Reading: An Introduction," *Representations* 108 (Fall
2009): 1–21.

28. Charles R. Lyons and James C. Lyons, "Anna Deavere Smith: Perspectives on Her Performance within the Context of Critical Theory," *Journal of
Dramatic Theory and Criticism* 9, no. 1 (1994): 47.

29. Martin and Smith, "Anna Deavere Smith," 56.

30. Susan Dominus, "Can Anna Deavere Smith's One-Woman Play about Health Care Bring Other Voices to the Debate?" *New York Times Magazine,* October 4, 2009.

31. Susan Dominus, "The Health Care Monologues," *New York Times Magazine,* September 30, 2009, accessed January 7, 2017, http://www.nytimes.com/2009/10/04/magazine/04smith-t.html

32. Gregory Jay, "Other People's Holocausts: Trauma, Empathy, and Justice in Anna Deavere Smith's 'Fires in the Mirror,'" *Contemporary Literature* 48, no. 1 (2007): 119–49.

33. Quoted in Attilio Favorini, "Fires in the Mirror: Crown Heights, Brooklyn, and Other Identities," *Theatre Journal* 48, no. 1 (1996): 105.

34. Martin and Smith, "Anna Deavere Smith," 57.

35. David Levin, "Choreographer's Opera: Bodies, Voices, and Meaning in Pina Bausch's Production of C. W. Gluck's *Orpheus and Eurydice,*" Albert Wertheim Seminar in Performance, Indiana University, 2012. A version of this lecture can be viewed at "David Levin, Choreographer's Opera," *The Mellon School of Theater and Performance Research at Harvard University,* http://thschool.fas.harvard.edu/icb/icb.do?keyword=k76089&panel=icb.pagecontent1163139%3Ar%241%3Ffr%3D21%26perPage%3D20%26sort%3D&pageid=icb.page386654&pageContentId=icb.pagecontent1163139&view=watch.do&viewParam_entry=80327&state=maximize#a_icb_pagecontent1163139

36. W. B. Worthen, "'The Written Troubles of the 'Brain,'" *Theatre Journal* 64, no. 1 (2012): 95.

37. D. J. Hopkins, "*Sleep No More.* Review," *Theatre Journal* 64, no. 2 (2012): 269–71.

38. W. B. Worthen, "'The Written Troubles of the 'Brain,'" *Theatre Journal* 64, no. 1 (2012): 87.

39. Hopkins, "*Sleep No More,*" 270.

40. Hilton Als, "Shadow and Act," *The New Yorker,* May 2, 2011.

41. Worthen, "'The Written Troubles of the Brain,'" 84. For an interesting argument that "immersive" theater and the "emancipated spectator" are not new ideas, see Marvin Carlson, "Immersive Theatre and the Reception Process," *Forum Modernes Theater* 27, nos. 1–2 (2012): 17–24.

42. Ibid., 91.

43. Ibid., 89.

44. Ibid.

45. Nicholas Rand Moschovakis, "Topicality and Conceptual Blending: *Titus Andronicus* and the Case of William Hacket," *College Literature* 33, no. 1 (2006): 127–50.

46. Hopkins, "*Sleep No More*," 271.

47. Als, "Shadow and Act."

Chapter 4

1. Stephen Hilgartner, *Science on Stage: Expert Advice as Public Drama* (Stanford, CA: Stanford University Press, 2000), 6.

2. Alexander Todorov, Anesu Mandisodza, Amir Goren, and Crystal Hall, "Inferences of Competence from Faces Predict Election Outcomes," *Science* 308, no. 5728 (10 Jun 2005): 1623–26.

3. Nicholas O. Rule, Jonathan B. Freeman, Joseph M. Moran, John D. E. Gabrieli, Reginald B. Adams Jr., and Nalini Ambady, "Voting Behavior Is Reflected in Amygdala Response across Cultures," *Social Cognitive and Affective Neuroscience* 5, nos. 2–3 (2010): 349–55.

4. Drew Westen, Pavel S. Blagov, Keith Harenski, Clint Kilts, and Stephan Hamann, "Neural Bases of Motivated Reasoning: An fMRI Study of Emotional Constraints on Partisan Political Judgment in the 2004 U.S. Presidential Election," *Journal of Cognitive Neuroscience* 18, no. 11 (2006): 1947–58. Weston is the author of *The Political Brain: The Role of Emotion in Deciding the Fate of the Nation* (New York: Perseus Books, 2007).

5. http://www.themarketingarm.com/, accessed February 26, 2015.

6. "Who Makes the List of Trustworthiness?" *NPR*, February 14, 2015, http://www.npr.org/2015/02/14/386227424/who-makes-the-list-of-trustworthiness

7. Ta-Nehisi Coates argues that it was racism that drove white voters to the polls in 2016 in his essay, "The First White President: The Foundation of Donald Trump's Presidency is the Negation of Barack Obama's Legacy" *The Atlantic*, October 2017.

8. Melena Ryzik, "What It's Really Like to Work in Hollywood (*If You're Not a Straight White Man)," *New York Times*, February 24, 2016, accessed February 19, 2016, http://www.nytimes.com/interactive/2016/02/24/arts/hollywood-diversity-inclusion.html. The documentary *Casting By*, directed by Tom Donahue, tells a similar story about the casting of Danny Glover for *Lethal Weapon* (1987). When casting director Marion Dougherty suggest-

ed Glover for the part of Roger Murtaugh opposite Mel Gibson as Martin Riggs, the director (Richard Donner) said "but he's black." Later the director admitted that the script "didn't say color" and when he assumed that thus the two characters were white, "it was like a nail in my heart. I'm bigoted. I didn't see it. [This moment] changed my life in casting, but more important it changed my life in reality." Tom Donahue, *Casting By*, HBO Documentaries, 2013.

9. Brandi Wilkins Catanese, *The Problem of the Color[blind]: Racial Transgression and the Politics of Black Performance* (Ann Arbor: University of Michigan Press, 2011), 27.

10. Virginia Valian, *Why So Slow? The Advancement of Women* (Cambridge, MA: MIT Press, 1999), 11, 2.

11. Ibid., 131–32.

12. Ibid., 104.

13. Ibid., 323. Henry rallies his troops into battle, promising them that "the fewer men, the greater share of honor" (4.3.22).

14. Juliet Eilperin, "White House Women Want to Be in the Room Where It Happens," *Washington Post*, September 13, 2016, accessed January 8, 2017, https://www.washingtonpost.com/news/powerpost/wp/2016/09/13/white-house-women-are-now-in-the-room-where-it-happens/?utm_term=.63a473b68b2e

15. Alex Burns and Matt Flegenheimer, "Did You Miss the Presidential Debate? Here Are the Highlights," *New York Times*, September 26, 2016, accessed January 10, 2017, https://www.nytimes.com/2016/09/26/us/politics/presidential-debate.html?_r=0

16. Kelly Riddell, "Hillary Clinton Calls the Entire Nation Racist," *Washington Times*, September 26, 2016, accessed January 10, 2017, http://www.washingtontimes.com/news/2016/sep/26/hillary-clinton-calls-us-racist-debate/

17. Katherine Fung, "Geraldo Rivera: Trayvon Martin's 'Hoodie Is as Much Responsible for [His] Death as George Zimmerman,'" *Huffington Post*, March 23, 2012, accessed January 10, 2017, http://www.huffingtonpost.com/2012/03/23/geraldo-rivera-trayvon-martin-hoodie_n_1375080.html

18. Matt Williams, "Obama: Trayvon Martin Death a Tragedy that Must Be Fully Investigated," *The Guardian*, March 24, 2012, accessed January 10, 2017, https://www.theguardian.com/world/2012/mar/23/obama-trayvon-martin-tragedy

19. Ta-Nehisi Coates, "Fear of a Black President," *The Atlantic*, September

2012, accessed January 10, 2017, http://www.theatlantic.com/magazine/archive/2012/09/fear-of-a-black-president/309064/

20. Tiffany A. Ito, Geoffrey R. Urland, Eve Willadsen-Jensen, and Joshua Correll, "The Social Neuroscience of Stereotyping and Prejudice: Using Event-Related Brain Potentials to Study Social Perception," in *Social Neuroscience: People Thinking about Thinking People*, eds. John T. Cacioppo, Penny S. Visser, and Cynthia L. Pickett (Cambridge, MA: MIT Press, 2006), 198.

21. Patrick Colm Hogan, *Affective Narratology: The Emotional Structure of Stories* (Lincoln: University of Nebraska Press, 2011), 1, 24.

22. Ibid., 242. See also Suzanne Keen, "A Theory of Narrative Empathy," *Narrative* 14, no. 3 (2006): 207–36.

23. "Michigan State Rep Barred from Speaking after 'Vagina' Comments," *NPR*, June 17, 2012, accessed February 2, 2015, http://www.npr.org/sections/thetwo-way/2012/06/14/155059849/michigan-state-rep-barred-from-speaking-after-vagina-comments

24. Most of the speech can be heard at "Rep. Lisa Brown Speaks Out against House Attack on Women's Health," YouTube video, https://www.youtube.com/watch?v=7eRyQi-o9MA I am grateful to Kate Babbitt for her reading of Brown's radical role-shift at the end of the speech.

25. Lisa Brown, "Lisa Brown: Silenced for Saying (Shock!) 'Vagina,'" *CNN*, June 21, 2012, accessed February 2, 2015, http://www.cnn.com/2012/06/21/opinion/brown-kicked-out-for-saying-vagina/

26. Kim Solga, *Violence against Women in Early Modern Performance: Invisible Acts* (New York: Palgrave Macmillan, 2009), 32.

27. Ibid., 33.

28. Ibid., 39.

29. Jill Bond, "Columbia Rape Victim Gets 'Collective Carry' Help Carrying Her Mattress," *Blue Nation Review*, September 11, 2014, accessed February 9, 2015, http://archives.bluenationreview.com/columbia-rape-victim-gets-collective-carry-help-carrying-mattress/ See also Cathy Young, "Flawed Narratives, Perfect Victims, and the Columbia Rape Allegations: Can Reviving the Old Myth that Women Never Lie Serve Justice in Any Way?" *Reason.com*, February 9, 2015, accessed February 9, 2015, http://reason.com/archives/2015/02/09/flawed-narratives-perfect-victims-and-th

30. Kate Taylor, "Columbia Settles with Student Cast as a Rapist in Mattress Art Project, *The New York Times*, July 14, 2017, accessed July 14, 2017, https://www.nytimes.com/2017/07/14/nyregion/columbia-settles-with-student-cast-as-a-rapist-in-mattress-art-proect.html?_r=0.

Chapter 5

1. Streep gave a master class in the Department of Theatre, Drama, and Contemporary Dance at Indiana University in 2014.

2. R. Darren Gobert, *The Mind-Body Stage: Passion and Interaction in the Cartesian Theater* (Stanford, CA: Stanford University Press, 2013), 86–87.

3. Ibid., 5.

4. Ibid, 12, 89, and 131.

5. Ibid., 106–7.

6. Ibid., 113.

7. For an argument about how a similar effect occurs in Shakespeare's metatheatrical moments, see Amy Cook, "King of Shadows: Early Modern Characters and Actors," *Shakespeare and Consciousness*, eds. Paul Budra and Clifford Werier (London: Palgrave Macmillan, 2016); Robert Weimann, "The Actor-Character in 'Secretly Open' Action: Doubly Encoded Personation on Shakepseare's Stage" *Shakespeare and Character: Theory, History, Performance, and Theatrical Persons*, eds. Paul Yachnin and Jessica Slights (Palgrave Macmillan, 2009), 177–96; and Paul Yachnin and Myrna Wyatt Selkirk, "Metatheater and the Performance of Character in *The Winter's Tale*," *Shakespeare and Character: Theory, History, Performance, and Theatrical Persons*, eds. Paul Yachnin and Jessica Slights (Palgrave Macmillan, 2009), 139–57.

8. Laura Otis, *Membranes: Metaphors of Invasion in Nineteenth-Century Literature, Science, and Politics* (Baltimore, MD: Johns Hopkins University Press, 2000), 27.

9. Ibid., 4, 9.

10. Ibid., 174.

11. Ibid.

12. Bruce McConachie, *American Theater in the Culture of the Cold War: Producing and Contesting Containment, 1947–1962* (Iowa City: University of Iowa Press, 2003), 115–19.

13. Ibid., 52.

14. Ibid., 207.

15. Ralf Remshardt, "*War Horse*, and: *Stovepipe* (Review)," *Theatre Journal* 62, no. 2 (2010): 273.

16. For more on emotion and empathy in the theater, see Amy Cook, "For Hecuba or for Hamlet: Rethinking Emotion and Empathy in the Theatre," *Journal of Dramatic Theory and Criticism* 25, no. 2 (2011): 71–87. See also Suzanne Keen, "A Theory of Narrative Empathy," *Narrative* 14, no. 3 (2006):

207–36. Bruce McConachie also critiques Coleridge's "willing suspension of disbelief" (New York: Palgrave Macmillan, 2008).

17. Samuel Taylor Coleridge, *Biographia Literaria*, http://www.gutenberg. org/files/6081/6081-h/6081-h.htm, accessed online, February 17, 2017.

18. Richard J. Gerrig and David N. Rapp, "Psychologcal Processes Underlying Literary Impact," *Poetics Today* 25, no. 2 (2004): 270.

19. I recognize that I'm metaphorically separating these two here in radical opposition to my belief in the centrality of emotions and the body in what we traditionally think of as "the mind."

20. Jill Bennett, *Empathic Vision: Affect, Trauma, and Contemporary Art* (Stanford, CA: Stanford University Press, 2005), 43.

21. Wanda Strukus, "Mining the Gap: Physically Integrated Performance and Kinesthetic Empathy," *Journal of Dramatic Theory and Criticism* 25, no. 2 (2011): 91.

22. Ibid., 92. She specifically cites Beatrice Calvo-Merino, C. Jola, D. E. Glaser, and P. Haggard, "Towards a Sensorimotor Aesthetics of Performing Art," *Consciousness and Cognition* 17, no. 3 (September 2008): 911–22 and Matthew Reason and Dee Reynolds, "Kinesthesia, Empathy, and Related Pleasures: An Inquiry into Audience Experiences of Watching Dance," *Dance Research Journal* 42, no. 2 (2010): 49–75.

23. Ibid., 95.

24. Ibid., 93.

25. Ibid., 94. Citing "Wheelchair Dancer," "Glee," Wheelchair Dancer Blog 13 November 2009, Web. http://cripwheels.blogspot.com/

26. Remshardt, "*War Horse* and *Stovepipe* (Review)," 273.

27. "Handspring Puppet Co.: The Genius Puppetry Behind *War Horse*," *TED.com*, March 2011, accessed June 2011, http://www.ted.com/talks/handpring_puppet_co_the_genius_puppetry_behind_war_horse

28. Andy Clark, *Supersizing the Mind: Embodiment, Action, and Cognitive Extension* (New York: Oxford University Press, 2008), 78.

29. Edwin Hutchins, "The Cultural Ecosystem of Human Cognition," *Philosophical Philosophy*. 27, no. 1 (2014): 36.

30. "Michael K. Williams Asks: Am I Typecast? #QuestionAnswers." To see this video, go to: https://www.youtube.com/watch?v=STkh15nZ1uA

31. Rosamond Rhodes, "Introduction: Looking Back and Looking Forward, in *The Human Microbiome: Ethical, Legal and Social Concerns*, eds. Rosamond Rhodes, Nada Gligorov, and Abraham Paul Schwab (New York: Oxford University Press, 2013), 2.

Bibliography

Akindele, Toni. "The Comedian Took to Twitter When No Designer Would Dress Her for the Premiere of Her Upcoming *Ghostbusters* Reboot," *Essence*, June 29, 2016.

Als, Hilton. "Shadow and Act," *The New Yorker*, May 2, 2011.

Anderson, Emily Hodgson. "Celebrity Shylock," *PMLA* 126, no. 4 (2011).

Auslander, Philip. *Performing Glam Rock: Gender and Theatricality in Popular Music* (Ann Arbor: University of Michigan Press, 2006).

Baron-Cohen, Simon. *Mindblindness: An Essay on Autism and Theory of Mind* (Cambridge, MA: MIT Press, 1995).

Bate, Jonathan, ed. *Titus Andronicus* (London: Routledge, 1995).

Barron, James. "Public Lives," *New York Times*, April 25, 2000, B2.

Bell, Sue. "The Force Awakens but What Happened to Carrie Fisher's Face?" Midlifexpress.com.

Bennett, Jill. *Empathic Vision: Affect, Trauma, and Contemporary Art* (Stanford, CA: Stanford University Press, 2005).

Bergen, Benjamin K. *Louder Than Words: The New Science of How the Mind Makes Meaning* (New York: Basic, 2012).

Best, Stephen and Sharon Marcus, "Surface Reading: An Introduction," *Representations* 108 (Fall 2009).

Billington, Michael. "Julius Caesar: Review," *The Guardian*, December 4, 2013, accessed May 31, 2016.

Blair, Rhonda and Amy Cook, eds. *Theatre, Cognition Performance: Language, Bodies, Ecology* (New York: Methuen, 2016).

Blair, Rhonda. *The Actor, Image, and Action: Acting and Cognitive Neuroscience* (New York: Routledge, 2008).

Bolens, Guillemette. *The Style of Gestures: Embodiment and Cognition in Literary Narrative* (Baltimore, MD: Johns Hopkins University Press, 2012).

Bond, Jill. "Columbia Rape Victim Gets 'Collective Carry' Help Carrying Her Mattress," *Blue Nation Review*, September 11, 2014.

Boone, Joseph A. and Nancy J. Vickers, "Introduction: Celebrity Rites," *PMLA* 126, no. 4 (2011).

Brantley, Ben. "Threesome to Tantalize and Behold: Daniel Craig and Rachel Weisz Star in 'Betrayal' on Broadway," *New York Times*, October 27, 2013.

Brantley, Ben. "Review: In 'Hamilton,' Lin-Manuel Miranda Forges Democracy through Rap," *New York Times*, February 16, 2015.

Brantley, Ben. "Review: 'Henry IV,' Donmar Warehouse's All-Female Version," *New York Times*, November 11, 2015.

Braudy, Leo. *The Frenzy of Renown: Fame and Its History* (New York: Oxford University Press, 1986).

Brustein, Robert and August Wilson, "Subsidized Separatism: Responses to 'The Ground on Which I Stand,'" *American Theatre*, October 1996.

Burns, Alex and Matt Flegenheimer, "Did You Miss the Presidential Debate? Here Are the Highlights," *New York Times*, September 26, 2016.

Butler, Judith. *Excitable Speech: A Politics of the Performative* (New York: Routledge, 1997).

Calvo-Merino, Beatrice, C. Jola, D. E. Glaser, and P. Haggard, "Towards a Sensorimotor Aesthetics of Performing Art," *Consciousness and Cognition* 17, no. 3 (September 2008): 911–22.

Carey, Benedict. "How Nonsense Sharpens the Intellect," *New York Times*, October 5, 2009.

Carlson, Marvin. *The Haunted Stage: The Theatre as Memory Machine* (Ann Arbor: University of Michigan Press, 2001).

Casting By. Directed by Tom Donahue. 2013. Los Angeles, CA: HBO Documentaries, DVD.

Catanese, Brandi Wilkins. *The Problem of the Color[Blind]: Racial Transgression and the Politics of Black Performance* (Ann Arbor: University of Michigan Press, 2011).

Clark, Andy. *Supersizing the Mind: Embodiment, Action, and Cognitive Extension* (New York: Oxford University Press, 2008).

Charnes, Linda. *Notorious Identity: Materializing the Subject in Shakespeare* (Cambridge, MA: Harvard University Press, 1993).

Clark, Graeme. "Tropic Thunder: The Stars Speak," *The Spinning Image*, accessed November 28, 2016.

Collins-Hughes, Laura. "Review: 'Awake and Sing!,' a Depression-Era Family Drama," *New York Times*, July 20, 2015.

Coates, Ta-Nehisi. "Fear of a Black President," *The Atlantic*, September 2012.

Coates, Ta-Nehisi. "The First White President: The Foundation of Donald Trump's Presidency is the Negation of Barack Obama's Legacy," *The Atlantic*, October 2012.

Cook, Amy. "Bodied Forth: A Cognitive Scientific Approach to Performance

Analysis," in *The Oxford Handbook of Dance and Theater*, ed. Nadine George Graves (Oxford: Oxford University Press, 2015).

Cook, Amy. "King of Shadows: Early Modern Characters and Actors," in *Shakespeare and Consciousness*, ed. Paul Budra and Clifford Werrier (New York: Palgrave Macmillan, 2016).

Cook, Amy. "For Hecuba or for Hamlet: Rethinking Emotion and Empathy in the Theatre," *Journal of Dramatic Theory and Criticism* 25, no. 2 (2011): 71–87.

Cook, Amy. *Shakespearean Neuroplay: Reinvigorating the Study of Dramatic Texts and Performance through Cognitive Science* (New York: Palgrave Macmillan, 2010).

Cook, Amy. "Staging Nothing: *Hamlet* and Cognitive Science,"SubStance 35, no. 2, 2006.

Dancygier, Barbara. *The Language of Stories* (Cambridge, UK: Cambridge University Press, 2012).

Dancygier, Barbara. "Multimodality and Theatre: Material Objects, Bodies and Language," in *Theatre, Performance and Cognition: Languages, Bodies and Ecologies*, eds. Rhonda Blair and Amy Cook (London: Methuen, 2016).

Dargis, Manohla. Review of 'Where the Wild Things Are' (2009), "Some of His Best Friends Are Beasts," *New York Times*. Published October 15, 2009. Accessed January 8, 2015.

Dyer, Richard. *Heavenly Bodies: Film Stars and Society* (New York: St. Martin's Press, 1986).

Eilperin, Juliet. "White House Women Want to Be in the Room Where It Happens," *Washington Post*, September 13, 2016.

Elam, Keir. "'In What Chapter of His Bosom? Reading Shakespeare's Bodies," in *Alternative Shakespeares, vol. 2*, ed. Terence Hawkes (London: Routledge, 1996).

Ellis, Hadyn D. and Michael B. Lewis, "Capgras Delusion: A Window on Face Recognition," *Trends in Cognitive Sciences* 5, no. 4 (2001).

Emigh, John. "Minding Bodies: Demons, Masks, Archetypes, and the Limits of Culture," *Journal of Dramatic Theory and Criticism* 25, no. 2 (2011).

Ensler, Eve. *The Vagina Monologues* (New York: Villard, 1998).

Fauconnier, Gilles. "Compression and Emergent Structure," *Language and Linguistics* 6, no. 4 (2005): 534.

Fauconnier, Gilles. *Mental Spaces: Aspects of Meaning Construction in Natural Language* (Cambridge: Cambridge University Press, 1985).

Fauconnier, Gilles and Mark Turner. *The Way We Think: Conceptual Blending and the Mind's Hidden Complexities* (New York: Basic Books, 2002).

Freedberg, David and Vittorio Gallese. "Motion, Emotion and Empathy in Es-thetic Experience," *Trends in Cognitive Sciences*, 11 no. 5 (2007).

Freeman, Lisa A. *Character's Theater: Genre and Identity on the Eighteenth-Century English Stage* (Philadelphia: University of Pennsylvania Press, 2002), 8.

Fung, Katherine. "Geraldo Rivera: Trayvon Martin's 'Hoodie Is as Much Re-sponsible for [His] Death as George Zimmerman,'" *Huffington Post*, March 23, 2012.

Garber, Marjorie. *Vested Interests: Cross-Dressing & Cultural Anxiety* (New York: Routledge, 1992).

Gerrig, Richard J. and David N. Rapp. "Psychological Processes Underlying Lit-erary Impact," *Poetics Today* 25, no. 2 (2004).

Gerrig, Richard J., David N. Rapp, and David W. Allbritton. "The Construction of Literary Character: A View from Cognitive Psychology," *Style* 24 (Fall 1990).

Gibbs Jr., Raymond W. *Embodiment and Cognitive Science* (New York: Cambridge University Press, 2005).

Glenberg, Arthur M., M. Sato, L. Cattaneo, L. Riggio, D. Palumbo, et al. "Pro-cessing Abstract Language Modulates Motor System Activity," *Quarterly Journal of Experimental Psychology* 61, no. 6 (2008): 905–19.

Gobert, R. Darren. *The Mind-Body Stage: Passion and Interaction in the Cartesian Theater* (Stanford, CA: Stanford University Press, 2013).

Goldman, Alvin. "Imitation, Mind Reading, and Simulation," in *Perspectives on Imitation II*, eds. S. Hurley and N. Chater (Cambridge, MA: MIT Press, 2005).

Goodman, Tim. "Tim Goodman on James Gandolfini: 'You Couldn't Look Away from Him'" *The Hollywood Reporter*, posted at 6:08 p.m., June 19, 2013.

Goodwyn, Wade. "Former Texas Gov. Rick Perry Launches Second Presidential Run," *All Things Considered*, NPR, June 4, 2015, 4:33 p.m. EST.

Hall, Katori. "Playwright Reacts to the White Casting of MLK in *The Mountain-top*," *The Root*, November 9, 2015.

Hart, F. Elizabeth. "Matter, System, and Early Modern Studies: Outlines for a Materialist Linguistics," *Configurations* 6, no. 3 (1998): 313–14.

Hilgartner, Stephen. *Science on Stage: Expert Advice as Public Drama* (Stanford, CA: Stanford University Press, 2000).

Hodgdon, Barbara. "Replicating Richard: Body Doubles, Body Politics," *Theatre Journal* 50, no. 2 (1998).

Hogan, Patrick Colm. *Affective Narratology: The Emotional Structure of Stories* (Lincoln: University of Nebraska Press, 2011).

Hopkins, D. J. "*Sleep No More*. Review," *Theatre Journal* 64, no. 2 (2012): 269–71.

Hutchins, Edwin. "The Cultural Ecosystem of Human Cognition," *Philosophical Philosophy*, 27, no. 1 (2014).

Hutchins, Edwin. *Cognition in the Wild* (Cambridge, MA: MIT Press, 1995).

Hunter, Heidi. "She Was TOLD to Lose 35 Pounds! Carrie Fisher Reveals She Had to Drop a Substantial Amount of Weight Before Reprising Princess Leia Role in Star Wars: Episode VII," *Daily Mail*, May 16, 2014.

"Is There Any Lighthearted News?" *The Rush Limbaugh Show*, December 23, 2014.

Ito, Tiffany A., Geoffrey R. Urland, Eve Willadsen-Jensen, and Joshua Correll. "The Social Neuroscience of Stereotyping and Prejudice: Using Event-Related Brain Potentials to Study Social Perception," in *Social Neuroscience: People Thinking about Thinking People*, eds. John T. Cacioppo, Penny S. Visser, and Cynthia L. Pickett (Cambridge, MA: MIT Press, 2006).

Johnson, Mark. *The Meaning of the Body: Aesthetics of Human Understanding* (Chicago: University of Chicago Press, 2007).

Keen, Suzanne. "Readers' Temperaments and Fictional Character," *New Literary History* 42, no. 2 (2011).

Keen, Suzanne. "A Theory of Narrative Empathy," *Narrative* 14, no. 3 (2006): 207–36.

Kemp, Rick. *Embodied Acting: What Neuroscience Tells Us about Performance* (London: Routledge, 2012).

Kendt, Rob. *How They Cast It: An Insider's Look at Film and Television Casting* (Los Angeles: Lone Eagle Publishing, 2005).

Kirsh, David and Paul Maglio. "On Distinguishing Epistemic from Pragmatic Action," *Cognitive Science* 18, no. 4 (1994).

Krulwich, Robert. "Neuroscientists Battle Furiously over Jennifer Aniston," *Krulwich Wonders: Robert Krulwich on Science*, March 30, 2012.

Lakoff, George and Rafael Núñez. *Where Mathematics Come From: How the Embodied Mind Brings Mathematics Into Being* (New York: Basic Books, 2000).

Lakoff, George and Mark Johnson. *Philosophy in the Flesh: The Embodied Mind and Its Challenge to Western Thought* (New York: Basic Books, 1999).

Lakoff, George and Mark Johnson. *Metaphors We Live By* (Chicago: University of Chicago Press, 1980).

Lakoff, George and Mark Turner. *More Than Cool Reason: A Field Guide to Poetic Metaphor* (Chicago: University of Chicago Press, 1989).

Levith, Murray J. *What's in Shakespeare's Names?* (Hamden, CT: Archon Books, 1978).

Loofbourow, Lili. "The Many Faces of Tatiana Maslany," *New York Times Magazine*, April 2, 2015.

Lutterbie, John. *Toward a General Theory of Acting* (New York: Palgrave Macmillan, 2011).

Lyne, Raphael. *Shakespeare, Rhetoric and Cognition* (Cambridge, UK: Cambridge University Press, 2011).

Macnamara, John. *Names for Things: A Study of Human Learning* (Cambridge, MA: MIT Press, 1984).

Marcus, Sharon. "The Celebrity System circa 1879," unpublished talk, (Indiana University, September 13, 2013), 23.

Marcus, Sharon. "Salomé!! Sarah Bernhardt, Oscar Wilde, and the Drama of Celebrity," *PMLA* 126, no. 4 (2011).

Martin, Carol and Anna Deavere Smith. "Anna Deavere Smith: The Word Becomes You. An Interview," *TDR* 37, no. 4 (1993): 51.

Maslin, Janet. "More Things in 'Hamlet' Than Are Dreamt of in Other Adaptations" *New York Times*, December 25, 1996.

McConachie, Bruce. *Engaging Audiences: A Cognitive Approach to Spectating in the Theatre* (New York: Palgrave Macmillan, 2008).

McConachie, Bruce. "Falsifiable Theories for Theatre and Performance Studies," *Theatre Journal* 59, no. 4 (2007): 553–77.

McConachie, Bruce and F. Elizabeth Hart. *Performance and Cognition: Performance Studies and the Cognitive Turn* (London: Routledge, 2007).

McConachie, Bruce. *American Theater in the Culture of the Cold War: Producing and Contesting Containment, 1947–1962* (Iowa City: University of Iowa Press, 2003).

McKinley, Jesse. "'Monologues' Making Political Connection," *New York Times*, April 21, 2000.

McNulty, Charles. "Critic's Notebook: 'Hamilton's' Revolutionary Power Is in Its Hip-Hop Musical Numbers," *Los Angeles Times*, November 4, 2015.

Moschovakis, Nicholas Rand. "Topicality and Conceptual Blending: *Titus Andronicus* and The Case of William Hacket," *College Literature* 33, no. 1 (2006): 127–50.

Nelson, Havelock. "Dr. Dre: The Chronic," *Rolling Stone*, March 18, 1993.

Nussbaum, Emily. "Cheaper by the Dozen: Tatiana Maslany's Magnificent Sister Act, on 'Orphan Black,'" *The New Yorker*, April 28, 2014.

Otis, Laura. *Membranes: Metaphors of Invasion in Nineteenth-Century Literature, Science, and Politics* (Baltimore, MD: Johns Hopkins University Press, 2000).

Pao, Angela C. *No Safe Spaces: Re-Casting Race, Ethnicity, and Nationality in American Theater* (Ann Arbor: University of Michigan Press, 2010).

Pareles, Jon. "Critic's Notebook: Rappers Making Notoriety Pay Off," *New York Times*, October 31, 1995.

Parker, Ryan. "Carrie Fisher Responds to Criticism about Her Look in New 'Star Wars,' *The Hollywood Reporter*, December 29, 2015.

Peterson, Andrea. "The Switch: The Sony Pictures Hack, Explained," *Washington Post*, December 18, 2014.

Popken, Ben. "Royal Baby Name? 500-to-1 Odds on 'Macbeth'" *Today*, September 9, 2014.

Quian Quiroga, Rodrigo. "Searching for the Jennifer Aniston Neuron," *Scientific American*, February 1, 2013.

Quian Quiroga, Rodrigo, Itzhak Fried, and Christof Koch. "Brain Cells for Grandmother," *Scientific American* (February 2013): 3135.

Quinn, Michael. "Celebrity and the Semiotics of Acting," *New Theatre Quarterly* 22 (1990).

Ramachandran, V. S. and Sandra Blakeslee. *Phantoms in the Brain: Probing the Mysteries of the Human Mind* (New York: Quill William Morrow, 1998).

Ramscar, M., A. H. Smith, M. Dye, R. Futrell, P. Hendrix, R. H. Baayen, and R. Starr. "The 'Universal' Structure of Name Grammars and the Impact of Social Engineering on the Evolution of Natural Information Systems," in *Proceedings of the 35th Meeting of the Cognitive Science Society*, eds. M. Knauff, M. Pauen, N. Sebanz, and I. Wachsmuth (Berlin: Cognitive Science Society, 2013), 3246–47.

Reason, Matthew and Dee Reynolds. "Kinesthesia, Empathy, and Related Pleasures: An Inquiry into Audience Experiences of Watching Dance," *Dance Research Journal* 42, no. 2 (2010): 49–75.

Remshardt, Ralf. "*War Horse*, and: *Stovepipe* (Review)," *Theatre Journal* 62, no. 2 (2010): 273.

Rhodes, Rosamond. "Introduction: Looking Back and Looking Forward," in *The Human Microbiome: Ethical, Legal and Social Concerns*, eds. Rosamond Rhodes, Nada Gligorov, and Abraham Paul Schwab (New York: Oxford University Press, 2013).

Richards, I. A. *The Philosophy of Rhetoric* (New York: Oxford University Press, 1936), 96.

Riddell, Kelly. "Hillary Clinton Calls the Entire Nation Racist," *Washington Times*, September 26, 2016.

Roach, Joseph. *It* (Ann Arbor: University of Michigan Press, 2007).

Roach, Joseph. *Cities of the Dead: Circum-Atlantic Performance* (New York: Columbia University Press, 1996).

Roach, Joseph. "It," *Theatre Journal,* 56, no. 4 (Dec. 2004).

Robbins, Philip and Murat Aydede. *The Cambridge Handbook of Situated Cognition* (New York: Cambridge University Press, 2009).

Robson, David. "Kiki or Bouba? In Search of Language's Missing Link," *New Scientist* 2821, August 17, 2011.

Rokotnitz, Naomi. *Trusting Performance* (New York: Palgrave Macmillan, 2011).

Ross, Robin. "Rush Limbaugh Condemns Idris Elba as the Next Bond Because He's Black," *TV Guide, Today's News: Our Take,* December 25, 2014.

Rule, Nicholas O., Jonathan B. Freeman, Joseph M. Moran, John D. E. Gabrieli, Reginald B. Adams Jr., and Nalini Ambady. "Voting Behavior Is Reflected in Amygdala Response across Cultures," *Social Cognitive and Affective Neuroscience* 5, no. 2–3 (2010): 349–55.

Russell, Richard, Brad Duchaine, and Ken Nakayama. "Super-Recognizers: People with Extraordinary Face Recognition Ability," *Psychonomic Bulletin & Review* 16, no. 2 (2009): 252–57.

Ryzik, Melena. "What It's Really Like to Work in Hollywood (*If You're Not a Straight White Man)," *New York Times,* February 24, 2016.

Schell, Hester. *Casting Revealed: A Guide for Film Directors* (Studio City, CA: Michael Wiese Productions, 2010).

Shaughnessy, Nicola, ed. *Affective Performance and Cognitive Science: Body, Brain and Being* (London: Methuen, 2013).

Sherman, Howard. "What Does 'Hamilton' Tell Us about Race in Casting?" December 3, 2015.

Simonson, Robert. "Off-Bway's *Vagina Monologues* Nets Stars A-Plenty," *Playbill,* January 24, 2000, *Sleep No More.*

Solga, Kim. *Violence against Women in Early Modern Performance: Invisible Acts* (New York: Palgrave Macmillan, 2009).

Soloski, Alexis. "She'll Play the Jewish Mother, and Wants Other Asian-Americans to Get the Best Parts, Too," *New York Times,* June 25, 2015.

Staples, Brent. "The Politics of Gangsta Rap: A Music Celebrating Murder and Misogyny" Editorial Notebook. *New York Times.* Aug 27, 1993.

Starks, Lisa S. "The Displaced Body of Desire: Sexuality in Kenneth Branagh's *Hamlet,*" in *Shakespeare and Appropriation,* eds. Christy Desmet and Robert Jawyer (London: Routledge, 1999).

States, Bert O. "The Actor's Presence: Three Phenomenal Modes," in *Acting (Re) Considered: A Theoretical and Practical Guide,* 2nd ed., ed. Phillip B. Zarrilli (London: Routledge, 2002).

States, Bert O. *Hamlet and the Concept of Character* (Baltimore, MD: Johns Hopkins University Press, 1992).

States, Bert O. "The Anatomy of Dramatic Character," *Theatre Journal* 37, no. 1 (1985).

Steinmetz, Katie. "From Messiah to Hitler, What You Can and Cannot Name Your Child: A Judge's Order Calls Attention to Rules Governing Baby Names," *Time*, August 12, 2013.

Stern, Tiffany. *Making Shakespeare: From Stage to Page* (London: Routledge, 2004).

Stoppard, Tom. *Arcadia* (London: Faber and Faber, Inc., 1993).

Strukus, Wanda. "Mining the Gap: Physically Integrated Performance and Kinesthetic Empathy," *Journal of Dramatic Theory and Criticism* 25, no. 2 (2011).

Sweetser, Eve. "Blended Spaces and Performativity," *Cognitive Linguistics* 11, no. 3/4 (2000).

Terry, Ellen. *Four Lectures on Shakespeare*, ed. Christopher St. John (London: Martin Hopkinson Ltd, 1932).

Thompson, Ayanna. *Passing Strange: Shakespeare, Race, and Contemporary America* (New York: Oxford University Press, 2011).

Thompson, Ayanna. "'Ay, There's the Rub': Race and Performance Studies," in *New Directions in Renaissance Drama and Performance Studies*, ed. Sarah Werner (London: Palgrave Macmillan, 2010).

Todorov, Alexander, Anesu N. Mandisodza, Amir Goren, and Crystal C. Hall. "Inferences of Competence from Faces Predict Election Outcomes," *Science* 308, no. 5728 (2005).

Tran, Diep. "On the Rights of Playwrights and White Tears: Lloyd Suh and Katori Hall Offer the Latest Teaching Moments in Race-Conscious Casting," *American Theatre*, November 16, 2015.

Tribble, Evelyn. *Cognition in the Globe: Attention and Memory in Shakespeare's Theatre* (New York, Palgrave, 2011).

Tribble, Evelyn and John Sutton. "Cognitive Ecology as a Framework for Shakespearean Studies," *Shakespeare Studies* 39 (2011).

Turner, Mark. "Double-Scope Stories," *Narrative Theory and the Cognitive Sciences*, ed. David Herman. (CSLI, 2003): 17.

Turner, Mark. *The Literary Mind* (New York: Oxford University Press, 1996).

Valian, Virginia. *Why So Slow? The Advancement of Women* (Cambridge, MA: MIT Press, 1999).

Vasari, Giorgio. *Lives of the Artists*, trans. George Bull (New York: Penguin, 1971).

Vermeule, Blakey. *Why Do We Care about Literary Characters?* (Baltimore, MD: Johns Hopkins University Press, 2009).

Wakeman, Gregory. "How Much Weight Was Carrie Fisher Asked to Lose for Star Wars: The Force Awakens," *Cinemablend*, December 2016.

Weimann, Robert. "The Actor-Character in 'Secretly Open' Action: Doubly Encoded Personation on Shakespeare's Stage" *Shakespeare and Character: Theory, History, Performance, and Theatrical Persons*, eds. Paul Yachnin and Jessica Slights (Palgrave Macmillan, 2009), 177–96.

Westen, Drew, Pavel S. Blagov, Keith Harenski, Clint Kilts, and Stephan Hamann. "Neural Bases of Motivated Reasoning: An fMRI Study of Emotional Constraints on Partisan Political Judgment in the 2004 U.S. Presidential Election," *Journal of Cognitive Neuroscience* 18, no. 11 (2006): 1947–58.

Westen, Drew. *The Political Brain: The Role of Emotion in Deciding the Fate of the Nation* (New York: Perseus Books, 2007).

Williams, Lawrence E. and John A. Bargh. "Experiencing Physical Warmth Promotes Interpersonal Warmth," *Science* 322, no. 5901 (October 24, 2008): 606–6.

Williams, Matt. "Obama: Trayvon Martin Death a Tragedy that Must Be Fully Investigated," *The Guardian*, March 24, 2012.

Wilson, August. "The Ground on Which I Stand," *Callaloo*, 20, no. 3 (1997).

Worthen, W. B. "'The Written Troubles of the Brain': *Sleep No More* and the Space of Character," *Theatre Journal* 64, no. 1 (2012).

Yachnin, Paul and Myrna Wyatt Selkirk. "Metatheater and the Performance of Character in *The Winter's Tale*," *Shakespeare and Character: Theory, History, Performance, and Theatrical Persons*, eds. Paul Yachnin and Jessica Slights (Palgrave Macmillan, 2009), 139–57.

Young, Cathy. "Flawed Narratives, Perfect Victims, and the Columbia Rape Allegations: Can Reviving the Old Myth that Women Never Lie Serve Justice in Any Way?" *Reason.com*, February 9, 2015.

Zunshine, Lisa. *Why We Read Fiction: Theory of Mind and the Novel* (Columbus: Ohio State University Press, 2006).

Zunshine, Lisa. "Theory of Mind and Experimental Representations of Fictional Consciousness," *Narrative* 11, no. 3 (2003): 270–91.

Zwaan, Rolf A., Robert A. Stanfield, and Richard H. Yaxley. "Language Comprehenders Mentally Represent the Shapes of Objects," *Psychological Science*, 13, no. 2 (2002): 168–71.

Index

acting, 46, 73, 79, 111–13, 135–37; and celebrity, 44–46, 70, 73; and age 65; and talent, 70, 80–81; method, 111–12, 139
Allbritton, David W., 54
Allen, Colin, v
Allen, Tim, 73
Allen, Woody, 13
Anderson, Emily Hodgson, 63, 68
Aniston, Jennifer, 32, 60–61, 63
Arcadia (Tom Stoppard), 103–4
Auslander, Philip, 91
Awake and Sing! (Clifford Odets). *See* National Asian American Theater Company

Babbitt, Kate, v
Bates, Kathy, 83
Bausch, Pina, 115
Bell, Sue, 82–83
Bennett, Jill, 142
Bergen, Benjamin K., 17
Betterton, Thomas, 14
Betrayal (Harold Pinter), 70
Billington, Michael, 105–6
binding, 26–27, 60
Black, Lewis, 73
Blair, Rhonda, vi, 152n46, 155n67
Blakeslee, Sandra, 59–60
Bond, James, 3–5, 20, 27, 70
Boone, Joseph A., 15
Bowie, David, 91
Boyle, Susan, 15
Branagh, Kenneth, 39, 42, 44–49, 64, 74, 78
Brantley, Ben, 70, 85, 106,
Braudy, Leo, 66–7
Breithaupt, Fritz, v
Brown, Rep. Lisa, 131–34
Brustein, Robert, 84
Butler, Judith, 42, 95, 157n13

Candy, John, 83
Capgras delusion. *See* facial recognition
Carlson, Marvin, 12, 15, 170n41
casting; in animated films, 73; break-downs, 10–11; cameo, 47–49, 137, 140, 158n21; "color-blind," 5, 84–85, 90, 95, cross-gender, 95, 105–8, 111; counter casting, 95, 111, 135, 140, 143, 145, 147–48; directors, 2, 10–11; differently abled, 144; nontradition-al, 83, 89; and race, 5, 83–95; 114, 119, 121, 129; transformational, 122, 130–34
Casting Society of America, 9–10
categories and categorization, 27–31, 38, 51, 55, 57, 75, 95, 108, 122, 124–28, 130, 132, 140, 146
Catanese, Brandi Wilkins, 5, 84–85, 89–90, 126
celebrity, 2, 12–5, 39–45, 48–9, 66–70, 73–75
character, 6–9, 14–15, 38, 43–44, 115–120
Charnes, Linda, v, 68
Clark, Andy, 55–56, 102
Clooney, George, 3, 4, 63
Close, Chuck. *See* prosopagnosia
Close, Glenn, 40–41
Clinton, Hillary, 5, 124, 126–28
cognitive; ecology, 104; linguistics, 18–9, 103, 117–18; load or "shrift," 32, 38, 53, 55, 62, 70, 102, 130; "turn" in the humanities, 25–6, 30, 102–3; hunger or workout, 69–70,77
Coleridge, Samuel Taylor, 63, 141
compression, 20, 35, 39; and Polar Vortex example, 36–38
conceptual blending theory. *See* concep-tual integration theory
conceptual integration theory, 20–23, 25–26, 36–38, 56, 117–19; 132; and Bypass example, 21–22, 36

Printed and bound by CPI Group (UK) Ltd, Croydon, CR0 4YY

09/06/2025

14685633-0001